Courage and Information

Courage and Information
For Life With
Chronic Obstructive Pulmonary
Disease

The handbook for patients, families, and care givers
managing COPD
(emphysema, asthmatic bronchitis, or chronic bronchitis)

Second Edition

Rick Carter, Ph. D., Brooke Nicotra, M. D., and Jo-Von Tucker, COPD Patient

With Forewords by
Thomas Petty, M.D. and Brian Tiep, M.D.
And with a new section on Family Matters by
Richard Knowles, Ph.D., Brian L Tiep, M.D., and Jo-Von Tucker

NEW TECHNOLOGY PUBLISHING, INC.
ONSET, MASSACHUSETTS

Courage and Information For Life With
Chronic Obstructive Pulmonary Disease:
The handbook for patients, families, and care givers managing COPD
(emphysema, asthmatic bronchitis, or chronic bronchitis)

New Technology Publishing, Inc.
6 West Boulevard—POB 1737
Onset Massachusetts 02558 USA

www.newtechpub.com
www.HealthyResources.com
email: copd@newtechpub.com

Telephone:
508-291-1111
888-706-COPD
800-762-7632
FAX:
508-291-1704
800-452-7632

™

This second edition contains a new section based on material first published at www.HealthyResources.com as part of the Spring 2001 issue of COPD TODAY. Under the title of *Family Matters* is an essay, "Collaboration for Health," by Richard Knowles, Ph.D. and Brian L Tiep, MD and an open letter to families by Jo-Von Tucker.

Neither the authors nor the publisher is engaged in providing medical or professional services through the distribution or sale of this book. Persons with suspected or diagnosed Chronic Obstructive Pulmonary Disease or any other medical condition or health problem should consult with a physician and other qualified professionals for advice concerning their own treatment.

The authors and publisher are grateful for the right to copy illustrations and use materials which are credited at "Copyrights and Trademarks" on page 245. The following are trademarks of New Technology Publishing, Inc.: Healthy Resources™, www.HealthyResources.com™, COPD TODAY™, www.newtechpub.com™, the logo of the hand grasping the sun, Courage and Information™, Phantom of the Night™, Phantom Sleep Resources™.

2001 2002 2003 2004 / 10 9 8 7 6 5 4 3 2 1 0
ISBN 1-882431-07-3

Publisher's Cataloging-in-Publication
(Provided by Quality Books, Inc.)

Carter, Rick, 1951-
Courage and information for life with chronic obstructive pulmonary disease : the handbook for patients, families, and caregivers managing COPD (emphysema, asthmatic bronchitis, or chronic bronchitis) / Rick Carter, Brooke Nicotra, and Jo-Von Tucker ; with forewords by Thomas Petty and Brian Tiep ; and with a new section on Family matters by Richard Knowles, Brian L. Tiep, and Jo-Von Tucker. -- 2nd ed.
   p. cm.
Includes bibliographical references and index.
ISBN: 1-882431-07-3

1. Lungs--Diseases, Obstructive--Popular works.
I. Nicotra, Brooke. II. Tucker, Jo-Von. III. Title.
RC776.O3C37 2001   616.2'4
        QB101 - 200724

Dedication

Rick Carter

This book is dedicated to my wife Lynn and our three children Brian, Stephen, and Lauren for their ongoing understanding and support. A special debt of thanks is extended to Brooke Nicotra, MD, Brian Tiep, MD, and Robert Payne, MD for their concern, passion and willingness to help others and to the many patients we have all grown to know. A special acknowledgment is due Dr. Allen B. Cohen, a lung research pioneer who stimulated many research and clinical interests at the University of Texas Health Center at Tyler, Texas. Lastly, I would like to recognize my parents and teachers to whom I am indebted.

Brooke Nicotra

This book is dedicated to my patients over the years who taught me so much and were a source of joy to me. My children, Charlie and Susie, have been a great source of encouragement throughout. I am grateful to the wonderful nurses, especially Debbie Ippolito, and the respiratory personnel who supported me over the years.

Jo-Von Tucker

I dedicate this book to the members of the *Cape COPD Support Group,* a deeply caring, warm and wonderful group of very courageous friends!

My heartfelt thanks go to the two pulmonary specialists who have guided me, who provided enthusiastic direction, and under whose care I have found enormous security and aid: Dr. Chet Mohr of Hyannis, Massachusetts and Dr. Talmadge King, formerly of the National Jewish Medical and Research Center in Denver, Colorado, who is now at San Francisco General Hospital. My book is for them also... because their care has extended my life.

Contents

List of Figures

List of Tables

Foreword: Taking Charge of COPD

Dr. Brian Tiep, M.D.

COPD (chronic obstructive pulmonary disease) is most accurately described as being both chronic and progressive. Not only is it here to stay—it gets worse over time. A combination of chronic bronchitis, emphysema and some component of asthma, COPD is most frequently caused by long term exposure to tobacco smoke. In fact, it rarely occurs in people who have not had this exposure. No cure is yet available and we cannot repair destroyed lungs. On the basis of this information, many patients and their health care professionals alike may be tempted to give up, welcome inactivity, and allow the disease to take its natural course. However, inactivity leads to deconditioning. Deconditioning causes you to become short of breath upon minimal exertion. Hence, your natural response to your disease actually intensifies the corrosive impact of your disease. Also, COPD sets the stage for multiple sub-diseases like infections and water retention. Even minor respiratory infections can pack a big wallop. However, these are preventable and treatable. You can avoid or at least slow that natural course. For good control of your disease, you have to participate in its management. You must take charge.

Destructive living habits are the usual root cause of your disease; likewise, constructive living habits will enable you to adapt and enjoy a rich quality of life in spite of your disease. This is a lesson learned from 30 years of pulmonary rehabilitation. If you are still smoking or someone close to you smokes, take immediate steps to remove that source of toxic exposure from your life. People fortunate enough to participate in a pulmonary rehabilitation program learn that yielding to inactivity is disabling.

Giving up control is tantamount to handing your life over to your disease. Conversely, becoming active and taking charge is enabling. Daily exercise recruits your body's support by building endurance, strength and confidence and reducing shortness of breath. By gathering your inner strength, life becomes more rewarding. Owing to self management, people who undergo pulmonary rehabilitation are hospitalized less often. Some are able to go back to work, while others enjoy more active leisure pursuits. Even if you do not have the opportunity to participate in a formal pulmonary rehabilitation program, you can still use the principles to enrich your life and control your COPD.

A practical description of the disease process will shed some light on how it is possible for you to manage your disease and your life on a daily basis. You can conceive of your disease as a three layer process. The basic layer relates to your loss of lung function. This is what your disease is doing to your lungs. It causes you to become short of breath when you exert. It is important to understand that your lung disease has been slowly advancing over many years—even before you could perceive that a disease process was present. This is because your lungs are divinely designed to meet your needs during heavy exertion. Accordingly, you can lose a great deal of lung function before you begin to feel it; eventually, your advancing disease will catch up with you by limiting your exertion to progressively lower levels. Detection of COPD in its earliest stages can lead to effective early intervention. Once the disease is detected, it is crucial to promptly take charge and halt its progression.

The next layer is the complication layer. This layer typically surfaces as the disease becomes more advanced. Because of oxygen deprivation and various causes, other organs in your body are affected. Beyond this point your lung disease alters your whole body. For example, your heart, circulation and muscles become less effective in performing their functions. Also, the side effects of medications come into play. Good self care helps to minimize the impact of the complication layer.

The most dynamic and menacing layer is the exacerbation layer. An exacerbation is an acute flare-up of your COPD. Your weakened lung defenses render you particularly vulnerable to lung infections. When most of us get a cold, it is a nuisance or inconvenience and is usually not serious. When a person with COPD gets a cold, it can become serious. A cold may develop into bronchitis or pneumonia. Your bronchial passages become swollen and clogged with secretions that become infected. Infection can cause damage to your bronchial linings creating a safe haven for bacteria to grow. Aside from infection, you become more sensitive to respiratory irritants. Tobacco smoke, perfumes, paint fumes, barbeque smoke and cleaning solutions—previously well tolerated odors—may trigger an exacerbation. Again, your airways become swollen and blocked by secretions and your breathing is more difficult.

The exacerbation layer is the main cause of disability from COPD. Fortunately, it is also the layer that is most treatable. Exacerbations can be prevented. Avoiding toxins, paint fumes, hair sprays, infections and other causes of exacerbation along with vaccinations against the flu or specific types of pneumonia may make a difference. Avoiding physical contact with people who have colds or flu can prevent the spread of infection. Hand washing both by the giver and receiver will often prevent transmission of a cold. Good hand washing can be accomplished both in the home and out in public. When soap and running water are not available, newer hand cleaning products are convenient and effective substitutes.

In spite of the best preventative measures, exacerbations still occur. They can and should be treated well in their earliest stages. This means that you must become knowledgeable about your disease, do a regular self-check of your breathing status and respond promptly and effectively. Your self-check will detect any change in breathing status—the key is change. The change you are detecting could be an increase in shortness of breath, less ability to exert, change in cough and sputum amount or color, fluid retention or fever. When you detect a change indicating an exacerbation, you should immediately call your physician and also immediately follow your physician's prescribed course of action. Ideally, your physician will have prescribed medication for you to have in your medicine cabinet to be taken in the event of an exacerbation. A five to seven day pulse of prednisone and an antibiotic effective for your disease may be prescribed by your physician with specific instructions on their use. Also, you should ask your doctor about using higher doses of your inhaled medication during this period.

Waiting for several hours or days risks allowing the exacerbation to become more advanced and promote lung damage. When lung destruction occurs, your body must undergo a repair process that takes time and drains your energy; it becomes a lengthy recuperation. Thus, it is necessary for you to learn to recognize the exacerbation process in its earliest stages and immediately initiate your planned treatment. This concept is consistent with a general notion in medicine that we can treat almost any condition if we can catch it early enough.

In effect you are developing a collaboration or partnership with your physician. Thus, you have a set of responsibilities requiring some training to care for yourself on a daily basis. Your role is self management, which includes prevention, adherence to a medication schedule, effective self administration of your metered dose inhalers, regular exercise, and exacerbation management. Your physician's role is to provide direction in addition to the usual physician responsibilities like diagnosis and prescribing treatment. Communication between you and your physician is essential. When you call your physician with an exacerbation, be ready to report the changes in shortness of breath and your secretions, whether you are wheezing or tight, have a fever or increase in your weight. When you see your physician for a regular office visit, you should likewise bring a list of pertinent changes in your condition. Also, bring a list of medications and your questions. Your physician visit will be more effective.

Self management does not have to end when you have to be admitted to the hospital. You can participate in your care while in the hospital. If you are skilled in the use of your metered dose inhaler, you can be assigned by your physician to take doses in between your nebulizer treatments. Your physician may direct the respiratory therapist to monitor your safe and effective use of your metered dose inhaler. Your metered dose inhaler is just as effective as the pressure driven nebulizer if used properly. You can do some walking to keep up your level of conditioning in the hospital. Additionally, walking will help to mobilize your secretions. If needed, your physician may order physical therapy to assist you and insure your safety. You can learn to cough effectively, in order to clear your secretions. Thus you can help to open your airways and clear infection in cooperation with your physician, nurses, and therapists. While some physicians are open to such patient participation, others are not. I believe that we will be seeing greater patient participation in the future.

In this book, Doctors Carter and Nicotra, two leading experts in the fields of pulmonary medicine, pulmonary rehabilitation and exercise, present you with a lucid and comprehensive description of your disease and ways you can manage it. Along with this critical knowledge, you will learn how to accept the disease that will have so much impact on your life. You will learn about your medications, how they work, their side effects and the importance of adhering to a good medication schedule. Understanding and acceptance of the disease are the first steps in good disease management. You will learn coping skills, nutrition, and the unique value of maintaining an exercise program. With the knowledge these authors impart in a clear, concise and friendly fashion, you will be able to work intelligently and collaboratively with your physician.

The third author is a remarkable patient, Jo-Von Tucker, who eloquently describes COPD from her personal point of view. Her hard road to acceptance granted her the insight that eventually enabled her to adapt by designing a workable and fulfilling lifestyle. She points to her role in creating a patient support group and how helping others has enriched her life and carried her through hard times. Support groups help people who have been isolated and darkened by chronic illness. She describes her own success story with well-lit guideposts. She creates a repertoire of memories that assist her through the hard times. She effectively creates a road map to successful attitude management with a practical approach.

The overall message emanating from this book tells us that it is not only possible and feasible to participate in your medical management—it is downright necessary. You can and should live a quality and rich life. This is a book that you should share with your doctor just as doctors should share it with their patients. This book should also be shared with your HMO, so that they can better understand how your participation can lead to good cost-effective COPD disease management.

I congratulate all three authors on a job well done. This book will potentially touch the lives of 15 million people and their families victimized by this tobacco-related disease. Unlike most popular books on COPD, this book should be read by patients and their physicians and the entire health care system. As medicine is becoming more technical, this book can serve as a nifty source for physicians and patients to share the same concepts leading to effective patient-physician collaboration.

Foreword

By Thomas L. Petty, M.D.

All patients with chronic obstructive pulmonary disease (COPD) should become expert in their own health care management. They should understand the basic nature of their problem, its course and prognosis, and how modern treatment can help to reduce the symptoms and enhance the quality of life that lies ahead.

Their doctor should be their consultant, as well as their friend and counselor. The relationship between patient and doctor is a key to success. This book is written from two viewpoints—the customer and the treatment provider, giving a basis for collaboration.

COPD is primarily a smoker's disease, which clusters in families and worsens with age. As doctors have learned about the underlying processes which damage the airways and alveoli and have developed powerful therapeutic approaches, they are better able to improve the lives of patients diagnosed with COPD, even in advanced stages of disease. Our early work in pulmonary rehabilitation showed both improved quality of life and length of life. Our pioneering oxygen studies also resulted in improved survival and life quality. Today, most people with COPD live into their seventies or eighties, a normal life span. How one lives, however, is at least as important as how long one lives.

Coping with anxiety, depression, and shortness of breath during normal activities is a challenge. It is a fact that the patient is the only one who knows exactly how the disease translates into individual feelings of loss. But the enlightened patient, equipped with modern knowledge, can be the key member of the healthcare team, with the goal of lessening the impact of COPD. The goal of pulmonary rehabilitation is to prevent premature loss of quality of life.

We are entering a new era of prevention. The National Lung Health Education Program (NLHEP) aims to identify patients in incipient stages of disease, who are mostly smokers beginning to lose airflow. A simple device, known as a *spirometer*, measures both airflow and volume. This device should be present in all primary care physicians' offices. Early identification can lead to smoking cessation, which is the most important therapeutic intervention. New approaches to inflammation, as well as nutritional strategies appear to be valuable for early stages of disease.

The authors are to be congratulated for producing such a readable and informative book. Not only patients and their families, but healthcare professionals will benefit from reading this timely handbook.

Introduction

A Dialogue Between Physician and Patient

If you have COPD—Chronic Obstructive Pulmonary Disease, sometimes called Chronic Obstructive Lung Disease (COLD)—or if you care for or take care of someone who has COPD, we wrote this book for you. We are two medical experts and a successful COPD patient with hard-won experience. We explain, from your point of view, the conditions causing COPD, the available medical and surgical treatment options, and how your efforts can determine the outcome.

Dialogue, good communication between doctor and patient is fundamental for success in managing COPD. Dialogue enables you to communicate and collaborate with each other, and with other care givers, to assure the best possible results.

Why is the doctor-patient relationship so important? Medical treatment can provide the most benefit when the patient and the physician work together, when each listens to and respects the other, and when the patient takes responsibility for his or her health. This dialogue is a skill which must be learned by doctors and by patients. Therefore, this book is intended to help you manage COPD, to help you talk with your doctor, if you are a patient; and with your patients, if you are a doctor.

Clinical and scientific information was written by the professional team of Brooke Nicotra, M.D., a pulmonary lung specialist, and Rick Carter, Ph.D., an exercise physiologist who specializes in improving function in the body even when disease is present. Jo-Von Tucker provides her insights, experience, and techniques, drawn from her experience living with COPD.

This book includes a mixture of advice and experience, suggestions, tips and helpful tools for managing COPD.

Maintaining the Best Possible Quality of Life

Courage and Information for Life with Chronic Obstructive Pulmonary Disease is intended as a practical and flexible guide to help you, your family and friends. COPD is a term commonly applied to any or all of: emphysema, asthmatic bronchitis, and chronic bronchitis.

This book is designed for those with little medical knowledge of COPD, as well as for those with some medical background. It is based on recommendations from experts for diagnosis and treatment of COPD. We hope that it addresses the most important issues facing anyone with this disease.

COPD is not like most health problems. *Chronic* means long term, so it will not go away. While there is no cure for COPD, nor for the diseases of COPD, there are many things you and your caregivers can do to minimize the impact. Your best chance of living a full life in spite of COPD is to actively manage your own health care—but you need to learn how. As you are the main person responsible for managing your disease process, you must learn how to work with the guidance provided by your doctor, and use your own management skills, to form an effective partnership for a productive and active life. The things you do at home every day will affect your life and abilities in the years to come:

- You decide to avoid cigarette smoke and other irritants.
- You decide to routinely use your medications.
- You decide what and when to eat.
- You decide to exercise.

Because your part is so vital, you need good information, so this book provides the information you need, and references to other sources of information to enable you to live, and live well.

Getting the Best Care

Learn as much as you can about your disease and your medicines.

Ask questions. This book can help you decide which questions to ask, so write a list and take it with you when you see your doctor or other health care provider.

Give information. Tell your doctor what your symptoms have been since your last visit. Be honest. Tell your doctor if you have had a change in your normal daily activity level. Talk about your medications and bring these with you at each visit. Discuss problems and concerns about any aspect of your medical management. Review your goals and talk with your doctor about these goals.

Follow directions. Write down what you are supposed to do. Repeat back what you think your doctor wants you to do. Be clear on all instructions before you leave the office. Take your medicines, and if on supplemental oxygen, use each as they are prescribed. Do not vary. If the medicines are too expensive or they don't seem to be working, tell your doctor, there may be other solutions.

Keep your appointments. Remind yourself to keep all appointments with your physician even if you are feeling better. If you cannot make an appointment, notify your physician as much in advance as possible and if you need to, request to speak with the doctor's nurse.

Pulmonary Rehabilitation Programs

Pulmonary rehabilitation programs are available in many hospitals and rehab facilities in many countries. The programs are intended to educate people about lung disease, and to teach closely-supervised exercises to restore as much physical conditioning and muscle toning as possible. This education will significantly add to the quality of life of a person with COPD.

The rehab/education sessions may last for six to eight weeks or longer with two-hour sessions two or three times a week. One hour is usually reserved for active exercise and physical therapy, and one for education or psychological counseling to help you cope with COPD and its impact.

You probably need to be referred by your doctor, and go through tests to be accepted into a pulmonary rehab program.

Dr. Brian Tiep and Dr. Tom Petty, whose Forewords open this book, are two of the leaders of pulmonary rehabilitation. Dr. Petty is considered by many as the modern-day father of pulmonary medicine, a tireless educator and champion of innovation. Dr. Tiep is one of the nation's pioneers of specially-developed pulmonary rehab programs for COPD treatment. They, and other experts in this field, are strong proponents of the roles of exercise, fitness, education, and mental attitude in restoring quality of life.

Their work demonstrates enormous benefits to people who commit themselves to a rehab program, so more and more facilities for such care and treatment are springing up around the U.S. and elsewhere. Australia, for example, has an active and growing community of pulmonary rehab programs with strong lung-support groups.

If you are able to enroll in a rehabilitation program, you will find this book helpful during the course and after it ends. However, even if you are unable to participate in a formal rehabilitation program, you can use this book to help build your own program, working closely with your doctors and other health care professionals.

How to Use This Handbook

This book may be used in an individual program or group wellness program to manage COPD early, in hopes of preventing the physical and emotional debilitation which often occurs. In patients with moderate or severe disease, it is best used in the setting of a formal rehabilitation program, allowing the patient the benefit of trained professionals. This assures patient safety and maximum emotional support, as the patient moves through a challenging program. Further, professional attention and support may permit the patient to achieve a greater level of activity, if someone is monitoring them closely for any ill effects, mental or physical, as well as encouraging them through the rough times which inevitably occur.

Scientific, medical, or technical terms are defined the first time they are used. A *Glossary* on page 225 provides a list of terms and explanations. Definitions are written in plain English.

This book covers breathing, diseases affecting breathing, diagnosis, medical and surgical interventions, nutrition, exercise, and the impact of smoking and stopping smoking. There is also extensive information and guidance on how your own outlook and determination, and the support of your family and friends, can make a difference. We encourage you to learn as much as you can about your medical problem.

Some of the most common questions about COPD are answered at the beginning of the book.

We encourage you to work closely with your doctors, nurses, respiratory therapist, exercise specialist, and nutritionist. Together, you can create a solid management plan and carry it through.

Use the space on each page for notes, and take this book to your next visit with your doctor or other health professional to get the answers for your specific needs. This book is intended to guide you in working with your doctors and other health professionals. It cannot replace their professional knowledge and concern. Please pay special attention to specific hazards and dangers that are flagged by the **WARNING** heading.

Rick Carter, Brooke Nicotra, and Jo-Von Tucker

The Voice of Each Author

Because there are three authors, they sometimes speak together and sometimes separately. We have used different typographic styles for clarity. The type style in this paragraph represents all three authors or the two medical professionals.

The style of this paragraph represents the voice of Jo-Von Tucker, telling her personal experiences and ideas and her understanding of the whole range of healing concepts; in addition to her interpretation of the scientific-professional-medical. Her personal experience provides the voice and perspective of a person with COPD.

Jo-Von Tucker's personal journal and letter is presented in this style.

This typographic style indicates a comment by all.   *RC, BN, JVT*

This represents a comment by Rick Carter.   *RC*

This represents a comment by Brooke Nicotra.   *BN*

This represents a comment by Jo-Von Tucker.   *JVT*

Online resources

The publisher of this book, New Technology Publishing, Inc., will make available updates to this book on the World Wide Web. *Healthy Resources*™ will also provide access to discussions and support groups among people with COPD, news, and information affecting people with COPD, and selected products. <http://www.HealthyResources.com>[1]

---

1. References to the URL or universal resource locator address system of the World Wide Web are set off by angled brackets, thus: <http://>.

Courage and Information

1 Frequently Asked Questions

What is COPD?

Chronic obstructive pulmonary disease (COPD) and chronic obstructive lung disease (COLD) are terms that the medical profession uses for chronic bronchitis, asthmatic bronchitis, and emphysema. They share a common trait: persistent difficulty in getting the air to flow out of the lung normally. Although other diseases cause difficulty in breathing and may be considered as COPD, this book focuses on chronic bronchitis, asthmatic bronchitis, and emphysema.

What causes COPD?

One fact is certain: cigarette smoking is a major cause of both emphysema and chronic bronchitis. The irritants in tobacco smoke inflame and eventually weaken the lungs, making them more susceptible to damage by bacterial infection.

Eighty-two percent of those who die of COPD are smokers, and smokers are ten times more likely than non-smokers to die of the illness. Although many of the lung changes of COPD are permanent, improvement in symptoms and signs of disease often begins when you stop smoking.

Industrial pollutants may also be a factor in some cases of emphysema. Prolonged exposure to cadmium or certain airborne fibers favors the later development of lung disease. Emphysema is also caused by an inherited problem which affects how your body reacts to lung damage. When you inherit a low level of a chemical called alpha-1 antitrypsin your lungs are easily damaged. Emphysema can develop over the years and your lungs overreact to cigarette smoke and to infections.

How do I know if I have chronic obstructive lung or pulmonary disease?

The prominent features of chronic obstructive pulmonary disease are cough, unusual amounts of sputum, and shortness of breath, with constant fatigue. Next to coronary heart disease, COPD accounts for more severe disability and untimely deaths than any other health-related problem in the United States. According to The American Lung Association, 15.4 million Americans are affected with COPD.

Do I really need to quit smoking and will it help me at this late date?

Quitting smoking is the single most important thing that you can do. Following your doctor's advice is next most important. When you stop smoking the lung disease that is present remains, but the ongoing insult to your lungs is immediately removed. This removal of cigarette smoke and the harmful agents it contains, also eliminates carbon monoxide from your blood stream. A repair process starts. Sputum and coughing decrease, taste returns, and you begin to feel better. Some lung damage is permanent, but by stopping smoking the progress of disease slows or stops. As repair starts, the number of infections tends to diminish, your taste for food returns, along with many other positive outcomes.

If I stop smoking is there still a chance that lung cancer may develop?

Yes. Lung cancer is a response to many years of smoking. The good news is, the sooner you quit and the longer you lay off smoking, the lower your chances for developing lung cancer.

Is my lung disease just going to get worse and worse until I die?

COPD is not very predictable. Your disease may stay the same for many years, during which you can maintain the same level of activity without increased difficulty in breathing. Or your health may go steadily downhill, or start to go downhill after severe illness.

I already have lung disease. Why should I quit smoking?

COPD will probably get steadily worse if you continue to smoke. In fact, if your disease is severe and you continue to smoke, your doctor may be able to closely predict when you'll die, as progression is steady.

Are my relatives more likely to have COPD because I do?

Yes. The reasons why only some smokers develop COPD are not entirely clear, but they relate to genetic inheritance.

Does my spouse's continued smoking hurt me?

Yes, if you have to inhale their smoke. Some people who quit smoking are extremely sensitive, wheeze and become short of breath with smoke exposure. For others, continued smoke exposure can make the disease develop faster.

Am I likely to develop cancer because I have lung disease?

Yes you are. People who smoke and develop COPD are more likely to develop cancer that those who smoke and do not develop COPD. This is another reason why it is crucial to stop smoking.

The color or amount of sputum that I produce has changed. Should I see a doctor?

Changes in the amount or color of sputum (or *phlegm*, or *spit*) you produce may indicate infection. Watch these changes closely. If you feel they are getting worse, talk with your doctor.

How can I improve my cardiopulmonary (heart and lung) health?

Don't smoke. Follow good medical advice. Take your medications regularly. Eat well and drink plenty of liquids, especially water. Get lots of rest. With your doctor, develop a program of regular, energetic, aerobic exercise for a prescribed intensity, frequency, and length of time. When planning your program be sure to include the type or mode of exercise, i.e., walking, cycling, swimming, weight training, etc. Use weight training to tone muscles and add some strength. See *Exercise and Nutrition* on page 121.

I have lost several pounds in the past year and I was not overweight to begin with. Is this significant?

Weight loss in people with lung disease can be significant. It indicates that you are no longer eating enough calories. Talk with your doctor. You may want to try eating five to six smaller meals per day, to increase calories. Avoid drinking a lot of liquid just before your meal because this fills your stomach. If you get short of breath while eating you may need to use supplemental oxygen or increase the flow rate while eating. You can also change the way your foods are prepared, or add foods with more calories. See *Nutrition* on page 141.

I want to lose weight, how do I get started?

Weight loss is using more calories than you eat in a day. The quickest way is to combine a sensible diet with exercise. As a pound of fat is about 3500 calories, if you use an extra 500 calories per day it will take seven days to remove a pound of fat. Exercise will help a lot in losing fat. Your body composition changes as you replace fat with muscle. A standard bathroom scale may not give you useful information about fat loss. A scale measures everything in the body at one time and can't report separately on fat weight, muscle mass, bone weight, or body fluids.

I've got COPD and I'm tired and discouraged, so why should I learn about it? Why should I work so hard? It's only going to be downhill, and anyhow my doctors should just tell me what to do?...

By learning about the disease and taking charge of your treatment, you can actually feel better and have a better quality of life. True, the permanent damage to your lungs can't be repaired. But if you stop smoking, exercise, eat a proper diet, and use medications in a proactive way, you can feel stronger and do more each day. What you know can help you work with your doctor to improve your health. Even when the disease progresses, you can retain control over your treatment if you make plans in advance. So there is a lot you can do and the rewards can be exceptional.

Do not get discouraged by minor setbacks. They are to be expected in this disease. Remain focused on your long term goals and consistently work toward achieving them.

2 You and Your Doctors

The Devastation of the Diagnosis

My name is Jo-Von Tucker. In 1989, at the relatively young age of 52, I heard the doctor trying to explain to me that I was very sick. I was diagnosed with chronic obstructive pulmonary disease (COPD). I didn't know what it was, what it meant, or just how sick I was.

A case of pneumonia that I came down with while on vacation on St. Maarten, and that preceded the diagnosis of COPD, led me to see my internist, and later, a pulmonary specialist. It was not my first case of pneumonia, and I had a much more difficult time getting over this one. After three changes of antibiotics, and nearly four months, I had recovered enough to start a battery of tests to determine the extent of damage to my lungs. But I still felt tired, weak and had a lot of chest pain and a persistent cough.

I had flown from New York, where I lived, to Denver, Colorado to get a second opinion at the National Jewish Medical and Research Center (NJMRC). All of my records and computed tomography images (CAT scans) had been forwarded from a pulmonary specialist in New York (who had never mentioned chronic obstructive lung disease to me, although she had expressed an opinion that I might have lung cancer and/or pulmonary fibrosis).

In less than a week, the hospital in Denver accomplished more than had been done in New York in eight weeks. The original tests were all repeated, plus they added quite a few of their own. I had chosen to seek the work-up and second-opinion at National Jewish after much research, both through my pulmonologist in New York and on my own. I had sought information on those hospitals rated the highest in research and diagnostic procedures in lung disorders, as well as for prominence in their treatment programs. NJMRC had come out at the top of the list. My experiences there validate their reputation as one of the best pulmonary facilities in the country.

The doctor I was to see in Denver had ordered supplemental oxygen for me as soon as I arrived at the airport. This was partly because of the readings of a battery of pulmonary function tests in New York, and partly because of the altitude of Denver, the "mile high city." Being put on oxygen was scary.

I had been directed to Dr. Talmadge King because the diagnosis in New York included the possibility of pulmonary fibrosis (and/or lung cancer), as well as emphysema. The doctor in New York had indicated the need to do open-chest, very invasive lung surgery to ascertain my diagnosis. I had insisted on a second opinion at a facility with an excellent reputation in lung work. Thus the referral to National Jewish Medical Research Center.

Completely alone in a strange city, on oxygen, amid the frightening surroundings of a hospital, with the incredible stress of not knowing exactly what was wrong with me, I was taken in hand by Dr. King's nurse and assistant, S. Arlene Niccoli, who soothed my fears with great caring and concern. Her compassion helped me to maintain some semblance of composure. Dr. King explained all of the tests and their objectives. Arlene went over the schedule so that I'd know what to expect.

I don't remember very much about the last session with Dr. King, when he shared the results of the testing and gave me the diagnosis and prognosis. Dr. King was then Director of the Cohen Clinic at NJMRC, and not a part of the unit primarily responsible for diagnosis and treatment of COPD. He was very kind and gentle as he explained what COPD was, and what it meant to me as a patient.

The two-hour session went by in a blur. I believe I was in a state of shock on that last day at the hospital. What I vividly recall is finding myself back in my Denver suite, with no notion of how I got there, crying so hard that I must have alarmed the neighbors. Actually I think "wailing" is a more appropriate word. I had never cried so hard, sobs wrenching my whole body in spasms of grief and fear.

I had just been ever-so-gently told that the prognosis for my life was probably less than five years.

My Reaction to the Diagnosis

My first reaction to the diagnosis was flight. I wanted to run away from everything, from everyone, especially from the truth about my illness. Even though I knew, deep in my soul, that I was very sick, I kept hoping that they were all wrong.

The pulmonary staff at NJMRC wanted me to stay for two weeks of rehabilitation training, but I made a mistake. In my grief and fear, I bolted for home. I caught the next flight back to New York, and holed up in my apartment like a wounded bear. For days I railed against the world, against God, against my body that had betrayed me.

Somehow I made arrangements for oxygen equipment and liquid oxygen, having been told by Dr. King that I would need supplemental oxygen 24 hours a day for the rest of my life. I contacted a home health care company, provided the prescription and paperwork they requested, and set about learning to use it in between bouts of serious depression. I didn't emerge from my apartment for days. I ordered food from the local market, or just ordered in. I left strict instructions with my office that I was not to be disturbed, by anyone, for any reason.

For me, this was bizarre behavior. I was a successful consultant in direct marketing, had my own business that I had moved from Dallas, Texas to New York City a few years before. I had traveled all over the world, and was active and involved. I gave speeches and conducted seminars on catalog marketing in London, Copenhagen, Tokyo, Dublin and Paris. I was named Direct Marketing

Woman of the Year just six months before I was diagnosed with COPD. I consulted for companies such as Neiman Marcus, L.L. Bean, Walt Disney and many others. Much of my catalog consulting was in France and Ireland, so it was normal for me to walk around with my passport in my briefcase. I've flown by Concorde a dozen times or more.

My idea of a great vacation was riding elephants through the jungles of Nepal or bouncing along in a pop-top van over the plains of East Africa on a photographic safari. I've been hot-air-ballooning over Australia, and white-water-rafting over Level 7 rapids in the Himalayas. I swam with manta rays in Bora Bora, and played blackjack all night in Monte Carlo. And I've spent countless hours walking the river banks in Connemara, the rugged and uniquely lovely west coast of Ireland, my favorite spot in all the world.

Obviously, I do not possess a retiring personality. So the fact that I hid in my apartment for days on end gives a pretty good idea of my state of mind. This was the self-imposed isolation that most people with COPD go through. I felt my life begin to slip away. I now had a chronic illness, and would be disabled for the rest of my life. What I needed to hear most was encouragement, that I didn't have to face this alone. Support systems, including pulmonology and rehabilitation professionals, support groups, and other health-care systems could help me. But I reacted to the diagnosis the way most patients do. I isolated myself.

I truly thought that I was in the process of dying.

Stages of Acceptance

I now know that almost everyone who has been diagnosed with chronic illness goes through nine stages of acceptance or denial, action or inaction, related to the illness. You must deal with each stage individually, as each is the lead-in to the next stage toward acceptance. None can be skipped if the healing process is to build a foundation of strength. Those stages are:

1 Grief
2 Denial
3 Rage
4 Self pity
5 Depression
6 Fear
7 Frustration
8 Resignation and acceptance
9 Finally you will choose life over death.

Education is the key to survival. Learn everything there is to know about COPD and associated illnesses so you can move toward peace, and a quality of life that can be sustained. This will let you manage the illness, rather than it managing you.

Grieving

We all grieve in our own way when a loved one dies. Likewise, when you are told that your body is in the process of dying, your first reaction is probably crushing grief.

Get help right away.

I felt an extreme sense of loss, just like receiving news of the loss of a family member or close friend. It seemed an irretrievable loss. Even before I learned all of the ramifications of COPD I sensed that my life would never be the same.

After the initial shock, I settled into deep mourning for my body and my life as I had known it. I grieved for the things that I could no longer do. I grieved for the loss of good health and I grieved for the things I had taken for granted all my life. Tears flowed incessantly. I found it difficult to talk to my family, even though they were filled with concern. I had always been considered the strong one in the family, the problem-solver, the one everyone else turns to for guidance, or consolation, or help. But I was falling apart. Friends couldn't comfort me, and I found it impossible to offer comfort to them. I just had to mourn, confronted by my own vulnerability and mortality.

Grief permeated every pore. I wallowed in it for days. Each time I would try to emerge, my emotions would slap me back into a chasm of sadness and loss. It simply did not occur to me to consult a psychologist, probably because I was so completely overwhelmed, and also because I was unable to let anyone know how I was feeling. I do wish now that I had been able to reach out for help.

I was so afraid of leaning on my family and friends, of pulling them down with me, that I was not able to see how badly I needed help.

Your doctor or nurse may recommend someone to talk to and suggest ways to get help.   *RC*

No one should have to go through the grief stage alone. Go to a caring friend or mate, or a family member with enough sensitivity to be understanding and helpful. Or go to a professional, preferably a psychologist or clergy. Also, find a support group or Better Breathers Club. See *Organizations* on page 237 for leads to finding a support group.

Denial

Denial for me was an overriding belief that this couldn't be happening. There must be some kind of mistake. Maybe they erred in all those tests. Maybe I just had another really bad bout of bronchitis. Maybe this was just a very long, terribly-realistic nightmare from which I'd awaken... healthy.

Denial is a toughie, and a stage that many people never successfully work through. It is very difficult to accept that you have a life-threatening illness, particularly a disease that is progressive, that eventually will result in death.   *RC*

I have always been a good compensator and this illness presented me with another opportunity. About eight or nine months before I got really sick, I had great difficulty walking in Manhattan (which I have always loved doing), becoming badly short of breath and experiencing chest pain after only a few blocks. I convinced myself that I was just tired; too much work, not enough rest. I had quit smoking cigarettes a couple of years before, but I did put in very long hours at work, and my international travel was exhausting. I was involved with a long-term catalog project for clients in Ireland, and made more than 24 trips there in two years. Jet lag was my constant companion.

I had also gained some weight after stopping smoking, and I was quick to equate that problem with my shortness of breath. But deep down, I knew that there was more. A tiny bit of exertion left me totally breathless. I would bend to pick up something off the floor, only to be hit by a stabbing burst of chest pain that, quite literally, brought me to my knees. The exhaustion was more than tiredness. But I compensated, and denied to myself that something might be seriously wrong.

Such chest pain is unusual in uncomplicated COPD and may have been one reason for misdiagnosis by the original doctor.   *BN*

When I was due to leave on a badly-needed vacation to St. Maarten, I confided some vague concerns about my health to Tom, my best friend. He encouraged me to see a doctor right then, but I had far too much to do. As it turned out, this was the vacation from hell. Most of it was spent in bed with pneumonia.

Six months later I got the bad news. My denial after diagnosis was even worse than before the pneumonia. I just could not accept the fact that I had chronic illness. Not me. No way.

Reality began to set in when I read the information from National Jewish Medical Research Center: pamphlets on emphysema, bronchitis and asthma; booklets on breathing exercises; my test results; exercise rehabilitation notebooks and workbooks; nutrition plans; and lots more, including reading recommendations for books on COPD available at a library or book store.

I had bolted from NJMRC in Denver before they could put me through their intensive pulmonary rehab program. I understand now the importance of careful outpatient management of a COPD program. It can make a big difference between a functional, fulfilling life and a life of pulmonary disability. The people at National Jewish Medical could have taught me ways to cope with a life of illness. But I headed for the Denver airport, and begged the counter people at American Airlines to hastily arrange the supplemental oxygen I would need on a flight home. (They were very kind, and did accommodate me, even though a 2-week notice was normally required.) I headed back to New York to learn what was in store for me the hard way, by reading.

I realize now that I could have benefited enormously by enrolling in the rehabilitation program and being taught by NJMRC experts. I would have been provided with emotional counseling, as well. And, believe me, I sure could have used that.

Little by little, my state of denial began to slide as reality set in, leading to the next stage: rage.

Rage

Anger takes a terrible toll. It will make a sick person much sicker.

I find it hard now to believe that I am even capable of such seething rage as I experienced in the weeks following diagnosis. Part of the rage was self-directed. It was very hard to accept my own responsibility in the impairment of my lungs, because COPD is, in most instances, an avoidable disease. No one forced me to smoke cigarettes. No one forced me to *keep* smoking cigarettes, even when the surgeon general's warning began to appear on the packages. And my COPD had not been caused by environmental or hazardous pollution, nor by an inherited gene fault. If I hadn't smoked, I would not have this illness.

So many thoughts went through my head, thoughts of my own mortality, and thoughts about the kind of life I'd lived to this point. I had no regrets about my life in regard to my fellow human beings, or to animals, for that matter. I have lived my life following the Golden Rule, the "Do unto others" philosophy, a life of giving and sharing that is my nature. So I wondered "Why me?" What on earth have I ever done to deserve this? For a time I even found myself questioning my faith, feeling abandoned by my God. I had done nothing in my lifetime to warrant such a desertion. And I was angry.

During this stage, my symptoms worsened, and I went through a series of lung infections. I began to believe that the five-year prognosis was optimistic—that at the rate I was going, I'd never live to see a second year, much less five.

While I was relieved that I did not have lung cancer, lupus or pulmonary fibrosis, I had been diagnosed with moderately severe COPD, including emphysema, chronic bronchitis and asthma.

I needed extra oxygen and training and equipment to use it. The first few times I ventured out with my portable oxygen unit on my shoulder and the nasal cannula tubing draped across my face and into my nose, looks from passersby ranged from curious to horrified. I was sensitive, acutely aware of the reactions of people around me to my new equipment. The rage deepened, and I was hesitant to go out. But gradually, I learned that the price I was paying for holding onto my anger was far too high. I knew that I had to accept my fate and move on.

Self Pity

The funny thing about self pity is that you are completely in control of it. This is one state of mind you can change. You can indulge in it if you wish, or you can put a stop to it when you refuse to feed it and let it grow.

I began to sink from anger to despair, feeling sorry for myself as I walked a few blocks to my office, gasping and pulling my portable oxygen on a little wheeled cart. I felt every stare, heard every whisper, and saw revulsion everywhere I looked. Self pity was a most uncomfortable state for me, and I choked on it for a time, hating the way it made me look and feel. But this is not an emotion that I can endure for very long.

Depression and Isolation

Anyone who has a chronic illness or disease periodically goes through some depression. Depression slips up on you without notice, and a lot of work must be done in order to emerge.

Depression was one of the worst phases I went through. It felt like being mired in molasses, unable to move, with enormous pressure pushing down on my head like a giant fist. The inability to act, or react, was awful, and I felt paralyzed. I found myself wanting to sleep; just let my consciousness slip away, retreat from chronic illness.

Living through my own experiences, and having worked with people in my lung support group, I now believe this is more than just a passing phase or stage of acceptance. Depression may emerge at any time.   *JVT*

Each time I realized that I had lost an ability or physical capacity for something I had loved, I encountered depression. The worst episode for me (and it comes back periodically) was when I understood that the brain, as a major body organ, must receive adequate oxygen. Oxygen deprivation eventually destroys brain cells. I began to notice short-term memory loss. "Please, God, anything but my mind. I can learn to live without hearing, or sight, or the use of my arms or legs, but please God, not my brain."

Depression itself may cause memory loss. The regular use of oxygen as needed will lower the likelihood of brain damage from oxygen shortage as a result of COPD.

BN

Fortunately, the memory loss episodes have not worsened, but my first bout with depression was a difficult one. The other major cause of depression for me was anticipation of loss of independence. I knew that the illness was progressive, and that I would gradually lose the ability to do everything for myself. Self-esteem becomes eroded as you become more dependent on others for help with the chores of daily living, especially if you are an independent cuss like me.

The result of depression was more sickness, each infection in my lungs more devastating than the one before. Since I have a severe allergy to penicillin, I was prescribed several different drugs before an effective medication was found. Prednisone, an effective medication for treating the symptoms of COPD, can rob the body of calcium, and was not prescribed for me because I have osteoporosis.

I do believe in "mind over matter," to a large degree. The mind can exert enough control to lighten symptoms, to soothe and sometimes heal. Once I realized the toll that rage was taking on my already-damaged body, I began to want to work my way out of depression. I grew curious about COPD, and began to want to fight it. I know that this is what helped me begin a healthier existence, and a search for a quality of life that I feared had been lost.

Attitude can make a big difference in most situations. Any improvement can lead to a stabilized status, even in a progressive disease like emphysema. Curiosity about obstructive lung disease helped push me right out of depression and into a fight for my life.

Fear of the Unknown

Fear comes in many forms: of being unable to breathe, of the treatments, of getting sicker, of loss of independence.

Fear reigned supreme and bordered on paranoia. This was not a very pleasant way to live. I knew that I had to conquer fear in order to retain some quality of life. I was driven at this stage to learn everything that I could about obstructive lung disease and its treatment. I knew that there was no cure for COPD, but there had to be ways to improve what was left of my life. Knowledge seemed to be the key. I have always been able to deal with whatever life dealt me, as long as I knew what I faced.

I knew very little about chronic obstructive lung disease, except that I had been diagnosed with it. My fear came more from lack of knowledge about the disease and not knowing what my life would be like, at least what was left of it. It was fear of the unknown. I was afraid every day. Fear greeted me each morning as I opened my eyes. I had not yet adjusted to sleeping with the nasal cannula plugged into my face, so I awoke most mornings with the tubing wrapped several times around my body, or with the cannula having slipped out of my nose resulting in a major morning headache. I had nightmares about being strangled. I still have nightmares about drowning, even though I was a good swimmer and had no fear of water.

I heard myself beginning to talk like John Wayne, with the -- hesitation -- between words or phrases -- as I caught my -- breath. I felt that I was going downhill very fast, and that I wouldn't last very long. I was afraid of being exposed to everyday viral illnesses (still am) for fear of having them turn into a bout of bronchitis, or worse, pneumonia. So I started to avoid movie theaters, crowds in stores, waiting lines, crowded elevators. As time passed, I also learned that a simple sinus infection could drain into my lungs, creating a dangerous situation that could become bacterial, with resultant infection.

Frustration

The frustration of not being healthy, and of losing independence can be dealt with by educating yourself and keeping busy.

It didn't take me long to realize that there was not very much information about COPD, particularly for lay people. I went through the workbook materials and pamphlets from National Jewish Medical many times, learning more each time. But it wasn't enough. I needed more. The bookstores, even in New York City, had nothing for me. I had to get them to special-order one book that had been recommended by Dr. King, *Enjoying Life With Emphysema* by Dr. Petty. I was incensed at the title, outraged that the author was so flip with such a serious situation. I did benefit from many of Dr. Petty's suggestions, but I felt like saying "Easy for you to say," to the author, a pulmonary doctor, but who did not have COPD. There is a new version of Dr. Petty's book titled, *Enjoying Life with Chronic Obstructive Pulmonary Disease*. Dr. Petty is a renowned expert in the field of COPD, and I include his books in the "must read" category. For a list of these and other helpful titles, see *Bibliography* on page 233.

Frustrated at the lack of credible information, I saw an ad for a data search from Planetree Health Resource Center in San Francisco. It offered to conduct a personalized data search for articles and research materials on any illness or disease. The cost for the complete packet today is $100.

I commissioned the search, and received a thick packet of documents about a month later. It was well worth the price. Finally, I had at my fingertips all of the latest information from medical journals, books, speeches by respected pulmonologists and research specialists, and much more. There was extensive information on treatments, both basic and experimental. There were reports on lung and heart/lung transplants.

There was also information about specific medications and their effects and side effects. I read and reread the entire packet like a starved person. Any spare time that I had from my work, I delved into research on COPD. Most of what was available had been written in medical terminology, not in lay terms, so it took some doing.

I believe that Jo-Von's ability to continue her usual activity, work, probably helped her through this stage. Keeping busy in some way is important as well for people who are unable to work.   *BN*

The more I learned, the less frustrated I was. Understanding the disease seemed to lead me more toward acceptance. I wasted less time on hopelessness and anger, and invested my now precious energy learning about obstructive lung illness, its treatment and outlook. I finally stopped "tilting at the wind," and started to use my strengths in a positive direction. Knowledge meant adjustment and acceptance, especially when I learned that many people were able to achieve a stabilized condition and to maintain a decent existence, even with COPD.

I remember being impressed by articles that reported the best results, stabilized, for those people who use supplemental oxygen 24 hours a day, as opposed to those who just use it at night or sporadically. I committed to religiously using oxygen, as prescribed. Cheating, or going without would only hurt me. Dr. King had prescribed supplemental oxygen 24 hours a day, seven days a week, and so it has been, for more than ten years.

It was a good feeling to begin to experience the dropping away of frustration and fear. It was encouraging to know that my resolve to live was strengthening, and each day that I worked on reading and study, I felt stronger and more like fighting for my life. There was a lot to learn. There still is, since new treatments and findings emerge all the time. My craving for more information lead me on a search for knowledge that helped me move from the role of patient/victim to that of person/survivor. Now look at me, nearly ten years later and writing about COPD for others.

Resignation, and Acceptance

Eventually you will find that making changes in your lifestyle, changing the way and the amount of things you do, even changing your means of earning a living, are the answers to fear and frustration. Dealing with things in practical ways is a sure path to living successfully with COPD.

It was a gradual move from resigning myself to the fact that I had COPD, to accepting all that went with it. I became resigned to not getting better, that my lungs can not regenerate. I began to accept what I could not change, but without the torment and fury that had been going on since I left Denver. I no longer blamed anyone else for my predicament. I had been a smoker for 30 years, albeit a relatively light one (pack and a half a day of Parliaments). I called my smoking "relatively light" simply because the doctors had said that I had a lot of emphysema for a little bit of smoking. Another factor was a light case, not crippling, of polio I contracted from oral polio vaccine when I was a young mother in my early twenties. This apparently left my lungs weakened, impaired, and undetected all those years. I had added insult to injury by smoking. I had stopped smoking two full years before I exhibited any symptoms of COPD!

Jo-Von had a 45 pack year (number-of-years times number-of-packs smoked daily) history of smoking. This is about average for people with COPD, though many smoke more, many less.   *BN*

It wasn't God's fault. I couldn't blame my parents or other family members. I couldn't even say it was the fault of my ex-husband. I am the one who made the decision to smoke, and who pushed myself with hard work to a dangerous level of low physical resistance. The smoking was an addiction, and one that I will pay for dearly, for the rest of my life. Now, let's get on with living it.

The most difficult part of acceptance had to do with lifestyle changes. I don't just mean the fact that I could no longer go trekking in the Himalayas. I mean, I would have to find another way to make a living. I loved being a direct marketer, and I was good at it. A lot of my work had been done for international clients. I had, early in my adult life, thrown myself passionately into my career and devoted enormous energy to it.

The prospect of losing my way of earning a living was dismal, scary, and caused me major stress. I couldn't hop a plane to Europe on a moment's notice anymore, and I had grave concerns about the way I would be perceived in business meetings with my portable oxygen unit and nasal cannula. There were other limitations: the portable oxygen tank was only good for about seven hours. It was like being on a short tether. I soon learned what a major hassle and logistic problem it can be to travel by air when you need supplemental oxygen all the time.

My experience traveling from Denver back to New York taught me some hard lessons. The airlines try to cooperate, but they need lead time to arrange for oxygen tanks on board. And they charge you $75 per flight segment for each cylinder of oxygen. See *Oxygen for Air Travel* on page 175 for more information.

Better methods of controlling oxygen flow allow you to use less oxygen. For example, with an oxygen conserving device (such as an Oxymizer™), one liter per minute may work as well as two liters per minute with a regular nasal cannula. This will increase the time a portable tank lasts. See *Supplemental Oxygen* on page 85. *BN*

As a busy New Yorker I had thought nothing of walking eight or ten blocks to a favorite restaurant, or of striking out to a cross-town appointment on foot, or of strolling Fifth Avenue. But walking, particularly uphill, is now difficult for me. And in New York City you can't fit a portable oxygen tank with its small cart in the back seat of a cab because the drivers always keep the seats pushed as far back as possible. Further, the pulmonary doctors all agreed that New York City was not a good place for me to live. One doctor said that if the air was so dirty that you could see it, it was too dirty for a lung patient to breathe it. The only place worse for me in the United States would have been Los Angeles.

Major changes were needed. Now I had to deal with managing this illness, comforting my family and friends, finding a new way to make a living at the age of 52, moving out of Manhattan, all in my spare time.

After an intense six months of study and comparisons of possible acquisitions, I decided to purchase a company already in the mail order business, and acquired Clambake Celebrations on Cape Cod. They packaged and shipped overnight delivery of live lobster clambake feasts. It seemed a good fit with my abilities.

Life Over Death: The Choice

Changed as it may be, you can live a rich and full life, even with COPD.

I had begun to realize that life could go on with COPD, and that it didn't have to be a matter of passive waiting for death. When I started to look around for a new way to support myself, and a different place to live, I chose life over death. There were many things that I could not do any more, but there were lots of things that I could still do, and maybe there were some new things for me to learn. My body didn't work very well anymore, but my brain seemed to be okay, at least so far.

Buying Clambake Celebrations was the best choice I had made in a long time. There were many challenges and I was a gal from Texas who knew nothing about lobsters except that I liked 'em (steamed, with drawn butter, please). I had to learn a lot, and quickly, but I loved the business, and dived into it with the same kind of passion I had always brought to my direct-marketing projects. I had a very good reason to push myself out of bed each day.

Living by the ocean where the air is clean and the sky sparkles deep blue—how it restored my battered soul. I start and end each day by the ocean, breathing deeply of the salty, moist Cape air. I even have my own car, allowing me independence in my daily activities. With a veritable new lease on life, I feel like The Little Engine That Could. Puff, puff, puff, I think I can, I think I can, an uphill battle, but one that I think I can handle after all.

Figure 1   Jo-Von Tucker at Clambake Celebrations

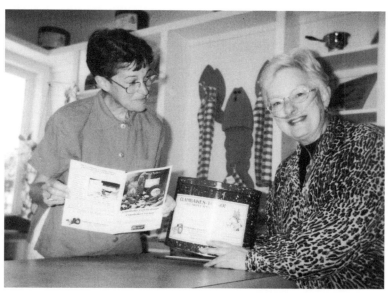

"Buying Clambake Celebrations was the best choice I had made in a long time." Jo-Von Tucker (right) explains the menu to Nancy Siegel, a visitor to Clambake Celebrations. Jo-Von and her staff provide succulent clam and lobster meals throughout the United States from clean, modern facilities behind an attractive Cape Cod storefront.

You and Your Doctor

Search for the Right Specialist

Finding the right 'fit' of a specialist is critical in dealing with a chronic illness. The price of one-on-one interviews with prospective doctors is worth it, to settle on the best doctor, with whom you have the best rapport, whose care will be instrumental in helping your fight. Do research on potential doctors just as you do research on everything about your illness. Information is a powerful weapon in your war chest for your fight with COPD.

Today in the United States, insurance plans direct you to specific physicians. If you have a choice, read the plan carefully before enrolling. Consider your situation, your present and future needs, physical access, hospital access, medical equipment provider access, and other issues. Do not select a plan simply because the monthly premium is a few dollars less.

As your chosen specialist will play a significant role in your life, you need to be sure that you have selected wisely, and that trust and rapport between you is high. Conduct interviews with prospective doctors. Let them know, up front, that this is what you have in mind for your first meeting. As with a request for a second opinion, a good doctor will not object. Understanding, good communication, and respect should be mutual between you and your doctor.

It is also a good idea to conduct your interviews before scheduling extensive tests. Ultimately, you'll save money by only having tests performed once, after you've chosen the specialist for your continuing care. You will, of course, be charged for the initial visit by each doctor you interview. It is fair, after all, to pay for their time and professional courtesy.

Unfortunately, such 'doctor shopping' may be very expensive. Many insurance companies have a very short list of pulmonary specialists to choose from. We suggest being frank with the doctor about your desire to have time to discuss both the medical problems and your own feelings. If you can't, get another doctor if at all possible.   *BN*

Doctor Interview Checklist

Here are a few points to include in your own list, when interviewing prospective doctors. Make it a rule to sit down right after your initial visit with a new doctor to document your interview list, so that your memory and impressions will be fresh.

1 Is a complete medical history taken before our first meeting?
2 Is our visit uninterrupted by phone calls or other distractions?
3 Does the doctor listen carefully to my symptoms before expressing an opinion or diagnosis?
4 Do I feel comfortable confiding in this doctor?
5 Can I clearly understand what this doctor is saying to me?
6 Am I impressed with his or her knowledge of the specialty?
7 Does this doctor really care about my state of health?
8 Was anything left undone in this first visit?
9 Is this the professional I wish to have looking after me?

Finding a Specialist In My New Home

Before leaving Manhattan for relocation to Cape Cod, I put in a call to Dr. King at National Jewish Medical Research Center in Denver. I wanted his advice about finding the right specialist in my new location. I was going to a place where I had no close friends, only acquaintances I had met through buying Clambake Celebrations.

Dr. King advised me to find a pulmonary specialist whose practice was on the Cape. Dr. King also reassured me about the general location of the Cape, that it is close to one of the world's great medical centers, Boston, with Massachusetts General, Brigham & Women's, New England Medical Center, and other fine hospital facilities. He felt it important to put major health care decisions in the hands of one doctor, preferably a lung specialist, because of the complexity of COPD and its overriding influence on a person's state of general health. He also felt it important for me to be physically close to my lung doctor, and suggested that I find a pulmonologist who would agree to be my primary care doctor.

Although not able to give me specific recommendations about doctors on the Cape, Dr. King suggested that I consult the company that had been supplying my oxygen on my visits to Cape Cod. I did so, and Cape & Islands Oxygen Company, which is owned and operated by Cape Cod Hospital, provided a list of qualified local doctors. With that list as a starting point, and after talking with other people in the community, I decided on Dr. Chester (Chet) Mohr. I found that Dr. Mohr is young, knowledgeable, progressive in his approach to lung disease treatment, and extremely nice and very caring in his relationships with his patients.

Dr. Mohr is one of those rare and special doctors who gives you his full attention for an unlimited amount of time, on each call or office visit. He has wonderful people skills, and communicates in plain language, never talking over my head in medical jargon, nor down to me as if I was three.

After my first visit with Dr. Mohr it was obvious that he was quite knowledgeable about COPD. I am constantly struck with how well he listens. Most of us are a bit shy when talking to a doctor, but I believe he hears the meaning behind the words. Our association is of mutual respect so that Dr. Mohr and I are partners in the management of my illness. He asks my opinions, and listens to my requests. During one of our first meetings, I told him I always wanted to be fully informed about my state of health, that nothing should ever be kept from me out of fear of my not being able to handle bad news. I told him that I could handle most anything, as long as I was being told the truth and was given complete information. We made a covenant to tell each other what needed to be said, good or bad. We have both kept that bargain, for the nine years I have been in his care.

Our doctor/patient relationship is so trusting that I am even comfortable relaying information over the telephone to Dr. Mohr's able nurse, Georgette. I know that she will concisely and accurately relate what I tell her to Dr. Mohr, and that I can expect a call back from him as soon as possible.

Whenever other specialists may be needed, as in the discovery of my diabetes, Dr. Mohr refers me to the proper doctor. I am under the care of an endocrinologist for diabetes, and copies of all my blood tests and work-ups are sent to Dr. Mohr simultaneously.

Partnership with Your Doctor

Good rapport with your doctor is vital.

It is a good idea to jot down your symptoms, so that you won't forget. Good doctors are not threatened by a person who walks into an examining room with a list of questions. It is easy to forget important things without a list, even when phoning your doctor.

It is also important to understand that doctors are people, too. They can make mistakes, and they can say the wrong things, just like the rest of us. But a doctor's word has usually been taken as the last word, unquestioned. It is called the *white coat syndrome*. A person's blood pressure may rise or fall, or the person may forget to relay important symptoms or information, or forget to ask questions just because the doctor's word is assumed to be final.

Your partnership with your doctor means that you accept your personal responsibility for taking an active role in managing your illness. You have the right to question a doctor's findings or recommendations. A questioning person is one who wants to learn as much as possible about their illness, and how to best manage it. At the very least, you need to understand the reasons for tests, the objectives, how soon results will be available, how literally results should be taken, and, most importantly, your options.

An excellent book is *Equal Partners* by Dr. Jody Heymann, a woman doctor who became critically ill, and was subjected to misunderstandings and misdiagnoses that lay people often encounter. Her book is recommended reading for anyone with chronic illness.

Equal Partners was written for doctors, patients, family members and other caregivers. In the book, Dr. Heymann relates her own life-threatening experience with serious illness and her frustration with the doctors who treated her. She reports how information was kept from her by some attending doctors, even though she is a practicing physician. Knowing that the situation is probably much worse for lay people, she offers in her book solid examples and suggestions for partnership in the treatment of your illness.

All of your symptoms are important to your doctor in making a diagnosis. Just a word for each symptom will be enough to jog your memory when you have your doctor or nurse on the phone. The time it takes to prepare a reminder list will serve you and your doctor well.

Prepare for the call by taking your temperature, taking your blood pressure if you have a monitor, and using your peak-flow meter to compare your lung function with your normal reading. (Unfortunately for many people with COPD, the peak flow is not very helpful. It is much more useful in asthma without COPD.) The same rules apply when planning a visit to your doctor's office. Make a brief list of issues to discuss, and include one-word reminders of symptoms to report. Your office visit will be much more satisfying if you arrive prepared and alert.

Symptoms Checklist

Add your own symptoms to this list below. All of this will help your doctor to diagnose.

❑ Shaky

❑ Color and amount of sputum

❑ Heavy or tight chest

❑ Fatigue

❑ Fever

❑ Headache

❑ Appetite loss

❑ Cough

❑ Aching muscles

❑ Difficulty breathing, short of breath

❑ Temperature: _____°F _____°C

❑ Blood pressure: _____/_____

❑ Distance walked at usual pace before stopping to rest:
_____(feet or yards; city blocks; etc.)

The Importance of Compliance

Open dialogue is an absolute necessity between doctor and patient. It will help you to understand what your doctor hopes to accomplish with prescribed treatment or medication. Ask questions, then follow instructions. Compliance means doing whatever your doctor recommends, and is necessary, if your doctor is to help you. A compliant patient receives better care and attention from a doctor, than a non-compliant patient. After all, it is terribly frustrating for a doctor to work with someone who disregards a carefully considered and educated treatment plan.

Non-compliance is not only frustrating for the doctor, it is unwise. Far better to openly discuss treatment, and ask questions than to simply not do what your doctor prescribes.

Compliance also means being conscientious about taking the doses of medications exactly when and how they are prescribed. No skipping, no stopping short, no doubling up, no substitutions. If the prescription bottle warns you to take a specific medication with food, do so for your own good.

Tell your doctor if the medication cost is preventing you from following instructions. Samples, medication substitutes, or discounts may be available for you.

RC, BN, JVT

One of the most common reasons people say that they don't follow the doctor's orders is money. If you are unable to afford the medications prescribed, this is a major barrier to compliance. You may have options that are less costly and equally beneficial. Use the list below to see if you can save money while becoming more compliant with your medication program:

- Explain to your physician your financial situation.
- Ask for generic drugs when possible.
- Price shop. Use the phone.
- For respiratory medications investigate bulk medicine rather than unit-dose medications.
- Ask your doctor if a different, less-expensive medication will do.
- Ask for free samples.
- In the United States, add-on (supplemental) insurance is available in addition to Medicare for extra cost.
- Another option may be the new Medicare HMO plan that covers drugs. However, do your homework because you lose some benefits with this plan, benefits that may be essential for you later.
- Ask your doctor about rebates and gifts from drug companies.
- Use a spacer with metered-dose inhalers (puffers) to receive maximum drug delivery. This will conserve medications and lower your monthly costs.
- Explore options with a social worker, if available in your area.

Discussion with your doctor will bring your values and life experiences to bear with your doctor's professional opinion and expertise in determining your treatment. A caring doctor will take into account a person's feelings and wishes. Then, after open discussion, if the doctor still prescribes the original treatment, comply to the best of your ability, or perhaps, find another doctor.

In *Equal Partners*, Dr. Heymann states that people who participate in their own care have greater satisfaction with their medical treatment, and that this can be measured in laboratory tests, as well as in decreased symptoms.

Involving people in their own care also results in significant savings over time. People often react to illness out of fear and insecurity, and may look for expensive tests and hospitalization as a result. Dialogue between doctor and patient can comfort and assure, eliminating or postponing the need for tests or hospital treatment.

I frequently push the boundaries on health treatment, never in a non-compliant way, but in a quest for new information on COPD. My doctor always listens patiently to whatever experimental test or surgical procedure I may have recently read about for obstructive airway disease treatment. Often, he has helped to get information on a new surgical procedure or experimental treatment and gives me statistical data on successes and failures. He is always open-minded and receptive to my inquiries, but is also quite conservative in deciding a course of action. A decision on whether or not to proceed is always mutual, based on his experience and findings, on his analysis of my medical history and current condition, and on my wishes as the patient.

Adequate Time for Office Visits, and Other Concerns

We all know how busy doctors are, and we are aware of the value of their time based on the charges for our office visits. And, too, we know that emergencies do come up, and must be dealt with. Taking all of that into account, we are still entitled to more than 10 minutes of our doctor's time when we have made an appointment.

Fortunately, with Dr. Mohr, I can always count on having an adequate amount of time. I come away from his office feeling reassured, and positive about his recommendations. But I fear that Dr. Chet Mohr is an exception.

According to my research, the average length of time a person in the U.S. receives for an office visit with their doctor, whether a specialist or a general practitioner, is 10 minutes. I do not believe that a doctor can hear what a person has to say about current health status, consider the person's history, do even a cursory exam, and come to a decision about prescribed treatment in 10 minutes.   *JVT*

Communicating With Your Doctor

If you are not getting the time you need for your doctor to understand your complaint, and to examine you before treatment is prescribed, I encourage you to stand up for your rights. Don't be intimidated by the fact that your doctor is a doctor. Although you will have your own way of asserting your right to more time with your doctor, make it known right then, at the time you feel you are being dismissed too soon. Tell the doctor, not the nurse, not the receptionist. Go to the source.

Whether a doctor's time has been scheduled too tightly, or an emergency has thrown the schedule off, people with appointments should not have a shortened visit. Just calmly and quietly tell your doctor that you need more time.

'Patience for patients' may apply if you are kept waiting. Try not to feel restless or neglected. Don't complain to the other people in the waiting room. They can't do anything about it and you'll only make everyone unhappy. Just be patient, and know that the doctor will see you as soon as possible. It is simple waiting-room etiquette, and courtesy. But once you are there in the examining room, ask for the time and attention that you need. At first your doctor may be a little uncomfortable with this approach, particularly if your doctor is used to being 'the boss,' at the top of the totem pole. While the doctor will always know more about how lungs work and about COPD than you do, you may know your own lungs better than your doctor.

Rehabilitation for COPD is a new concept in medicine. So after reading this book you may find yourself more aware of the benefits and methods of rehabilitation than your doctors.

To show that you are knowledgeable, you must do some basic work. One of the most important things to do is to quit smoking. No doctor will respect your knowledge if you argue about whether continued smoking is harming your lungs. At the very least, you must make the doctor aware that you know the importance of cigarette smoking in causing COPD. You must make it clear, if you have not stopped smoking, that you really want the doctor's help in doing so. See *Smoking* on page 105.

You must become familiar with your medicines and know as much as you can about them. Telling the doctor that you "have a pink inhaler and take two white pills" is not going to convince a busy doctor that you can manage your own disease.

Partnership between you and your doctor is through mutual trust. You need to follow the doctor's recommendations whenever possible. Although a realistic doctor knows that nobody follows every suggestion, if you don't do what the doctor orders, you must have a legitimate reason. In a time of unprecedented health care changes, you may be facing high medical bills and limited time with your doctor. It is extremely important that you understand your medical condition and speak knowledgeably so that you waste neither your time nor the doctor's. Your doctor can then rely on you as a more active partner in your own health care.

Your Responsibilities

Learn. Learn as much as you can about your disease and your medicines. This book is a start, but use the other sources of information suggested throughout the book, in the *Bibliography* on page 233, and in *Other Resources* on page 237.

Ask questions. Use this handbook to help decide which questions to ask.

Write lists. Take a list of issues and/or questions with you when you see your doctor or other health care provider.

Give information. Tell your doctor what your symptoms have been since your last visit. Be honest. Tell your doctor if you have had a change in your normal daily activity level. Talk about your medications and bring them with you at each visit. Discuss problems and concerns you have about any aspect of your medical management. Review your goals and talk with your doctor about them.

Follow directions. Write down what you are supposed to do. Repeat back what you think your doctor wants you to do, to be sure you heard correctly. Be clear on all instructions before you leave the office. Take your medicines as they are prescribed. Do not vary. If the medicines are too expensive or they don't seem to be working, tell your doctor, there may be other solutions.

Keep your appointments. Keep all appointments with your doctor even if you are feeling better. If you cannot make an appointment, notify your doctor as much in advance as possible and if you need to, request to speak with the doctor's nurse.

Your Doctor's Responsibilities

A physician's viewpoint: Brooke Nicotra, MD

Knowledgeable about lung disease in general and COPD in particular.

Diagnoses accurately.

Knows the possible complications, warns the patient, and prevents complications when possible.

Knows the accepted treatments for COPD, especially the different medications. This is a large area and usually requires a specialist in lung diseases. The many different medications have very different roles and may have permanent side-effects. A doctor cannot know every new "treatment" mentioned on the Internet or in a newspaper. Most of these have not even been published in a reputable medical source, much is not based on fact, and is often self-serving, meaning that the person publicizing it expects to make money.

Compassionate and patient with you over the years, as you learn about your disease and as it interferes with your life.

Is honest with you about what is likely to happen. Explains frightening and confusing things such as life support and respirators, if it seems you may need them.

Helps you make decisions about your life, using living wills and durable powers of attorney.

Tells you when he or she does not know the answer to your questions. Each person is unique and so is their disease. Doctors say "Nothing in medicine is 100% sure," so your doctor can only give you information about what is likely to happen based on knowledge and past experience.

Listens to your concerns and understands your need to communicate fears, loneliness, even economic problems related to the disease costs.

Supports you directly and refers you to other sources, for example, a rehabilitation program to suit your needs.

Is fair and straightforward with you about visit prices and other fees.

The office staff is professional, patient and empathic. They never forget that their job is to serve you, the patient.

A patient's viewpoint: Jo-Von Tucker

A physician's responsibility begins with the Hippocratic oath, to "First, do no harm..."

Listens when we describe symptoms and health concerns.

Diagnoses and prescribes treatment.

Fully explains the treatment plan, and makes sure that instructions are completely understood.

Prescribes follow-up care such as a phone call to the doctor's office after a certain period of time, and makes a follow-up appointment.

Discusses possible side-effects of medicines.

Encourages you to take an active roll in managing COPD.

Counsels on good and bad expectations and outcomes for COPD progression.

Provides sources for information on physiological and emotional changes that may occur.

Provides the message that life isn't over by discussing how to protect against exacerbations, and preserve wellness or relative stability of disease. See *The Way to Stay Stable* on page 82.

Behaves toward you as a human being in need of information, counseling, comforting, and possibly consoling.

An Open Letter from Jo-Von Tucker to the Doctor

Dear Doctor:

This letter is meant to say the things that I cannot always bring myself to say when I am in your office, and as I know many other people with COPD share my feelings, I speak on their behalf as well. Please bear with my attempt to explain the depth of my feelings about what may be a touchy subject.

This letter is about my critical concerns, and my innermost thoughts and feelings about my illness. It is my wish that my words will help you to help me, as you are the one delivering the bad news about the gravity of my situation.

I realize the huge responsibility that you bear, as you are, next to immediate family members, the most important person in my life. Most of us feel an almost tangible bond with you, relying heavily on you to guide us in effective treatments and illness management. You are the foundation of our support with your knowledge and professional expertise.

We need doctors who are able to relate to us and to the pain that we feel. We need to know that you care about us as individuals. We need you to have time for us when we need your attention. We need your reassurance that we'll be able to deal with the variety of problems that come with diagnosis of chronic illness and in helping us understand them. Our families, too, may need more from you than just hard, cold medical facts.

Dr. Greg Franchine of National Jewish Medical Research Center, states: "The person afflicted has to be a co-participant with the physician, and other resource people, thus achieving maximum control rather than a cure."

We need really good interpersonal skills from you, and all too often they are lacking.

You may resent the fact that we expect you to know all there is to know about our diseases, and at the same time expect a dimension of caring and involvement that you may not be willing or able to provide. But we who have chronic obstructive pulmonary disease ultimately must deal with the diagnosis, and with the fundamental changes in our lives. We must find an emotional balance that enables us to go on with our lives. We face anxiety and apprehension, particularly fueled by a lack of knowledge about our illnesses. We feel isolated from all those other people out there who don't have a chronic disease. And all of these intense feelings may also be laced with liberal portions of anger (at ourselves if we've been diagnosed with preventable diseases), and of inadequacy and helplessness.

People with chronic illnesses are faced with heavy demands on their psyches and their souls, as well as on their bodies. The shock that I felt as I sat with my doctor and heard him give me the devastating news that I was a victim of a progressive pulmonary disease is the shock that every person must bear with such a terrible diagnosis, although everyone reacts to it differently, depending upon their personality, their coping skills, and their illness. But one thing is for sure: all of us on the receiving end of a diagnosis of COPD have a serious need to find and maintain some measure of hope, along with a satisfactory self-image and some confidence to go forward.

I know that you, dear Doctor, must walk the fine line between truthful medical communication and personal feelings of a caring human being caught up in the grieving and suffering of your patient. Those intensely emotional diagnostic times must be very hard for you. I can surely understand why physicians have learned, over the years, to maintain a safe, clinical distance from the people who make up their practice. It can't be easy to have to tell someone that their life will be drastically altered, and radically shortened, by the ravages of a long-term disease. It has to be stressful.

As patients, we believe that it would be extraordinarily helpful if our doctors would understand that much of what is told to us at diagnosis is mired and lost in the shock of the moment. So much of what you tells us is not retained. It may be some time before the full impact takes effect. By realizing this, you may be able to provide us with important reading material that we can take home with us, and that we can begin to absorb on our own, in privacy.

Dr. Franchine looks at this as another set of coping mechanisms, or skills that people use in seeking relevant information, using their intellectual resources defensively. In other words, to paraphrase Dr. Franchine, knowledge relieves uncertainty and anxiety, even negative knowledge. By using our minds to seek reliable information, we can get control and become active participants in our own care.

So as well as sending us home with good reading material to help us learn about our illness, you should also realize that very soon we'll need more information from you. Please don't just send us away with another appointment in six months. Plan, instead, to help us right away, as we learn and adjust to the drastic changes required of us. Stagger several appointments relatively quickly after diagnosis, to check on our acceptance and progress, to help us as we struggle.

Some people, obviously, are able to get on with sound management of their illness much faster than others, while some become bogged down in depression, and may need counseling. You should be prepared to make a referral. Other people will move slower from the adjustment stage to acceptance, and it is entirely possible that close monitoring by you, their doctor, will bring them great comfort and speed their search for control and stability.

Do you know, Doctor, the degree of incapacitation and disability that a patient will suffer?

Do you have positive reinforcement to give us, with constructive suggestions to help us overcome some of our losses?

Can you help us deal with the stress of being chronically ill, perhaps by teaching us certain coping techniques?

Can you be sure that we are leaving your office armed with as much information and knowledge as we need to go face-to-face with disease and all of its discomfort and pain?

Can you recommend and refer us to a pulmonary rehabilitation program near our home? Are you aware of a support group and can you help us find it?

Can you recommend a book to read, one that will encourage us to keep fighting while being pragmatic about the disease and its unavoidable issues?

Most importantly, Doctor, please don't ever begin your statements with... "Well, for your age, you...". You have no idea how upsetting it is to hear you say that because of age, you will choose a less aggressive treatment program than you would for a younger person! You see, none of us really want to admit to ourselves that we are old. We don't feel old. We just feel sick. We read newspapers, and we are subjected to news reports on television. We know that recent studies have proven that in many cases physicians will take a much more moderate and conservative approach to treatment with patients who are 60 or older. We would prefer to believe that we will be given the same options for treatment as anyone else, regardless of age. We should at least have a say in the decision whether or not our illness or disease will be treated aggressively or with surgical options. Discuss it with us, and give us the respect that we give you.

We value your vital role in helping us manage disease. Yours is the strongest influence on our significantly-changed lives. So we ask for your understanding and consideration as we go through the process of completely reevaluating our life's priorities. It is a daunting project. With your help, we can move through acceptance, into compliance, coping, effective illness management and, hopefully, stability. With your help, we'll be able to accept courageously the challenge of chronic illness.

Respectfully,

Jo-Von Tucker, and all your other patients

3 Breathing and COPD

How We Breathe

The American Lung Association has, as their motto, "If You Can't Breathe, Nothing Else Matters.®" There is nothing more frightening than to not be able to breathe. Although COPD does make breathing difficult, you can learn to overcome fear and maximize your breathing. In order to understand COPD, its treatment and management, you need to understand some basics about how your body works, some basic physiology.

Your lungs pull air in, transferring the oxygen into your blood, where it is pumped by your heart to the rest of your body to provide oxygen and sending the blood back to your lungs where the carbon dioxide is pushed out by your lungs. Lung tissue does not regenerate, so loss of lung function is permanent. We can train other parts of our bodies to compensate for this loss, at least to some degree, but we cannot restore our lungs after significant damage from emphysema, chronic bronchitis and severe asthma.

The authors of *Shortness of Breath* point out that most people with breathing problems should become actively involved in their own health care, rather than passively receiving care from others.

This means that you need to learn all that you can about your illness and its symptoms, and try to learn about breathing exercises, medications and treatment. From this foundation will come an ability to cope with the disease, and important methods of holding onto, or regaining, quality of life.

If You Can't Breathe...

Breathing can't be taken for granted, especially by people with COPD. You need to realize how important breathing is to both physical and mental well-being.

I had my first encounter with a severe asthma attack, and was frightened nearly out of my wits, shortly after moving to Cape Cod. Fear turned the breathing problem into a full-fledged panic attack. This experience demonstrated more than anything else the wisdom of learning about COPD.

The asthma component of obstructive lung disease was one that had received the least amount of my attention and the fewest attempts at self-education. I had previously been plagued with bouts of bronchitis and pneumonia, and emphysema with its nagging and incessant *dyspnea*, or shortness of breath.

But in July of 1992 I was awakened about five o'clock in the morning after a hot, unbearably humid night by a dilly of a storm. Rain was falling in a steady, heavy downpour. Great blasts of thunder shook the house, lightning illuminated my bedroom as though it was midday instead of predawn. The electronic fire alarm was blasting away from the hall.

I ran around trying to figure out how to make that piercing siren stop. I closed the slider door onto the upper deck, lowered the window in the master bathroom, hoping to keep out some of the pressure and humidity from the storm. Then I rushed downstairs to shut windows and sliders. By this time, I was gasping for breath, just from lowering windows, shutting doors, and going down and back up the stairs to my bedroom.

The alarm stopped and I went back to bed, assuming that my breathing would calm down and return to normal. My inhalers (bronchodilators) were downstairs, and I must have fallen asleep very quickly.

About 45 minutes later, I woke up to realize that I was in trouble. I couldn't catch my breath. It was difficult even to sit up, and I struggled for a few minutes to get out of bed. It wasn't just shortness of breath—I couldn't breath! I put on a robe and made my way downstairs, going straight to my inhalers, both of them. But in my panic, I gulped at them much faster than I should have, allowing no time between puffs. I desperately needed help.

Be sure you know which inhaler to use in an emergency. The inhalers which help the most are the quick-acting bronchodilators like albuterol. See *Medications for COPD* on page 69.   *BN*

After about 15 minutes the inhalers should have begun to kick in and ease my labored breathing, but I was getting worse. I felt as though I was sucking air through a straw. As a hot beverage can ease shortness of breath, I made a pot of coffee, and tried to drink a cup. It didn't help.

In the bathroom mirror my face was ashen grey, my lips blue. This was enough to send me to dial 911. I gasped into the phone that I was a COPD patient, and that I couldn't breathe.

When The Eastham Fire Department paramedics and emergency medical technicians arrived minutes later, I was barely able to unlock the door for them. They commented on my deep-purple lips, asked a few questions, took my pulse, listened to my chest, and had me loaded into the ambulance within a couple more minutes. I was terrified.

As I was having chest pains, and feeling horribly constricted, the paramedics started an intravenous drip, and administered corticosteroid drugs through a nebulizer (breathing-medication machine) on the way to Cape Cod Hospital. I could hear the siren, but was aware of little else. I began to breathe easier before we reached the hospital, thanks to the fast action of the paramedics. At the Emergency Trauma Center, the doctors monitored oxygen levels in my blood and continued treatments for seven hours, checking vitals and oxygen saturation every 15 minutes or so.

My breathing and oxygen level improved, and I was allowed to go home later in the day. But the doctor warned me to get the proper amount of rest after such an episode, and told me that it would take me awhile to get over the insult to my body. My daughter took me home, still in my robe and nightgown.

It took me months to recover. At first I was as weak as a newborn kitten, unstable and fuzzy in my mind. I wasn't sure if I would ever be able to return to full-time work, or even get back most of my faculties. A lot of fear was involved in my recovery. I thought for a time that I might be dying.

In retrospect, if I had known more, I don't think I would have been as frightened, and I know I would have reached for help sooner. I just didn't know what was going on.

Later, Dr. Mohr said he was surprised that I hadn't suffered a previous acute asthma attack, and that I should be prepared for others as part of the COPD. Since then, I have done extensive study of the disease, and feel much better prepared. Next time, I'll know what is going on and when to call for help.

The Breathing System

Your breathing system includes your nose, mouth, a pair of lungs, the tubes or airway to the lungs, chest bones and muscles. Behind your nose are the warm, damp passages that join with the back of your mouth to form your throat. These passages clean the air as it goes through them. As air and food cross paths in the throat, a small flap of tissue called *epiglottis* closes the windpipe opening when you swallow, so food and liquid go down your *esophagus* (passage to the stomach), not into your lungs.

Figure 2   Healthy airway and lungs

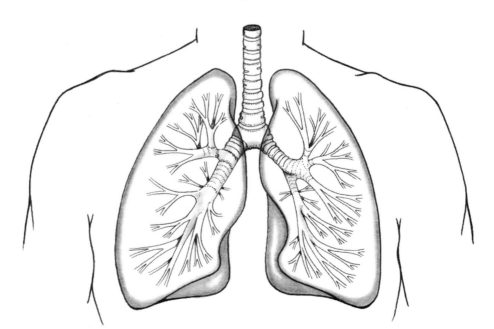

The airway is a series of tubes which start at the mouth like the trunk of a large, upside-down tree, then split into the right and left main bronchial tubes or *bronchi*. The bronchi branch down, as *bronchioles*, with each smaller than the one before.

The airway is a series of tubes which start at the mouth like the trunk of a large tree, then split into the right and left main bronchial tubes or *bronchi*. The bronchi branch down, as *bronchioles*, with each smaller than the one before. At the end of the bronchioles, like bunches of microscopic grapes, are millions of sack-like balloons, the *alveoli* or *alveolar sacs*, too small to see without a microscope. Oxygen (O_2) from the air crosses through the walls of the alveoli into the blood, which both takes up the oxygen from the air, and gives off a major waste product, carbon dioxide. The process of air traveling through the bronchi to the alveoli and crossing into the blood is called *respiration*.

Bronchial Tubes (Bronchi or Airways)

The bronchial tubes or airways are actually made up of a substance called *fibrous tissue* which is like skin. It can't stand up or keep its shape alone, but has to have support around it to stiffen it. This support is provided by *cartilage*. You can feel what cartilage is like by touching your ear or the front part of your nose; it's springy and holds its shape well.

Around the bronchial tubes are muscles. These are like the ones in your arms or legs, except that the bronchial muscles stay more relaxed and work automatically, so you don't have to think about them. Inside the lungs, the airways branch into smaller and smaller airways. These tiny airways are soft like cooked macaroni. Between the soft, floppy airways and the big rigid ones, all of the airways are wrapped in special muscles which can change the bore, or diameter of the airway by relaxing or contracting.

It is these muscles around the bronchial tubes which cramp or spasm when you have an acute asthma attack. Bronchodilator medications work by relaxing these muscle spasms, so the bronchial tubes can reopen.   *BN*

Figure 3   Healthy and diseased bronchial tubes

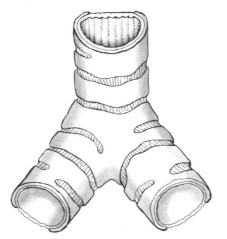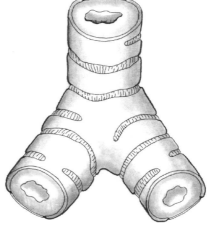

Healthy bronchial tubes have a large, open airway for normal breathing.

But bronchial tubes affected by bronchitis have only a very narrow airway, restricting breathing.

A soft velvet-like substance lines each airway, which is normally very smooth and slippery. This lining is made up of several different kinds of cells, the basic building blocks of the body. The lining cells of the bronchial tubes are called *epi-*

thelia, and protect the deeper layers, like paint on a wall. Some of these cells have *cilia*, tiny hairs which act like the oars in a racing boat. They all push together in one direction, then slide back quickly to get ready to beat again.

Mixed in among the cells with cilia are other glandular cells which make mucus. When irritated, these glandular cells pour out mucus, so that when you have a cold your nose fills, and even worse, if the bronchial tubes become irritated, inflammatory cells, which don't belong in the lung, are drawn down into the lung.

When your respiratory system is working well, you don't think about breathing unless you swim a mile or run a marathon, or climb a mountain. When the system is damaged, the muscles of the airways tighten up and squeeze the bronchial tubes, causing a cramp or spasm. The lining of the bronchi swells up, and the inflammatory cells rush in. Glands pour out mucus and the tiny cilia go in all directions at the wrong speed. You have bronchitis. If you're lucky, these structures will recover, the bronchitis will clear, and your system will return to normal. But if you've irritated the bronchial tubes too much, they will never recover and you develop chronic bronchitis. You cough, and unpleasant stuff comes up. Even worse, all that swelling and mucus and cramping causes you to wheeze and be short of breath.

Figure 4   Healthy and diseased cilia

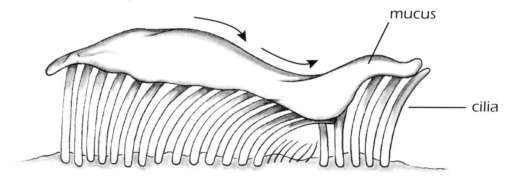

Some of the cells that line the bronchial tubes have cilia, tiny hairs which act like the oars in a row boat. They all push together in one direction, then slide back quickly to get ready to beat again. Mixed in among the cells with cilia are glandular cells which make mucus. The wave-like motion of the cilia moves the mucus away from the lungs and towards the mouth. The mucus traps foreign particles and carries them out of the airway, protecting the airway from infection and irritation.

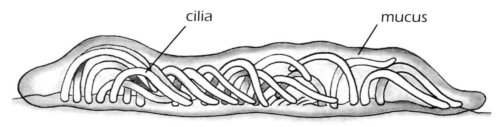

In bronchitis, the cilia are damaged, losing their ability to move the mucus while the cells that produce mucus have become irritated and produce too much mucus.

Normally the bronchial tubes are like a garden hose, with a narrow wall and plenty of room inside for the water to flow. But when your bronchi fill, they become like the hose half full of mud. The bronchial tubes fill with mucus and the muscles tighten up. The air can't flow through and you can't breathe normally.

In its mild form these unpleasant feelings become noticeable during exertion and thus the patient avoids exertion.   *RC*

Alveoli

The alveoli at the end of the bronchial tubes number in the millions. If all your alveoli were spread out flat, they would cover the surface of a tennis court. A healthy adult has about 300,000,000 alveoli in each lung. In the alveoli, the last branching of the airways, oxygen exchange really gets going. The walls of the alveoli are very thin, usually a single cell. The alveoli are found in clusters that are like a bunch of grapes. Each alveolus is surrounded by many capillaries and lymph vessels. The blood vessels and the lymph vessels run in the walls between the alveoli, forming a very large area of contact between the air and the fluids.

The problem is that there are so many alveoli, that you don't realize they are being damaged until about half of them are gone. And once they're gone, they never grow back. The remaining alveoli blow up further in an attempt to replace the losses, but it doesn't work. The blood vessels are destroyed, so that even if you can get air into the remaining alveoli, there aren't enough blood vessels to take up enough oxygen. Emphysema is a result of this destruction.

The Impact of Emphysema

Emphysema causes you to be short of breath because the air going in and out doesn't do enough good. Enough oxygen doesn't get into the body. So all that extra breathing with the remaining, inflated alveoli, is wasted. You get worn out with useless effort. Exercise makes things even worse, and there's nothing the doctor can do to restore the damaged alveoli.

So how do people with emphysema breathe at all? Well emphysema is a spotty disease. It may damage or destroy one area of lung and leave alone the area right next to it. Most of the useful work of breathing is done in the areas which are still normal or close to normal. How much normal lung is left is what determines how much you can do and how long you will live. This makes it crucial to protect every bit that's left after you become aware that you have emphysema.

The Balance of the Respiratory System

Your lungs and your chest cavity are both lined with a thin slippery membrane called a *pleura,* that allows lungs and chest wall to slide easily past each other as you breathe. Normally, there is no air or fluid between the two sets of pleura except the tiny bit of fluid greasing their movements. The linings have sensitive nerves.

Figure 5   Healthy and emphysemic alveoli

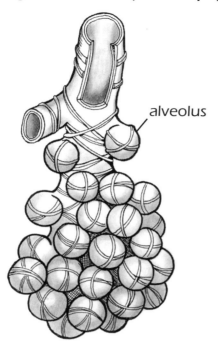

alveolus

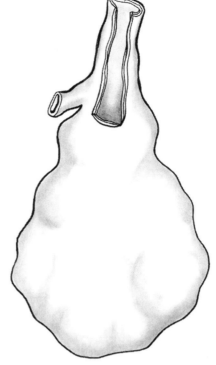

Oxygen exchange takes place in the alveoli, the last branching of the airways. The walls of the alveoli are very thin, usually a single cell, allowing oxygen and carbon dioxide to pass between the air and the blood. The exterior of the alveoli is like a bunch of grapes. Each alveolus is wrapped in an elastic membrane that expands and contracts with each breath.

But in emphysema the walls of the individual alveoli have broken down and what remains is an enlarged, flabby envelope that doesn't fully expand and contract with each breath. See another view, *Interior of healthy and emphysemic alveoli* on page 42. See also *Oxygen and carbon dioxide pass between the air and the blood* on page 37.

The most important protective covering for the lungs, however, is the chest cage, which includes all the ribs, the spine or backbone, and the place where the ribs join in front, the sternum or breastbone. All these parts of bone or cartilage are mostly held together by rib muscles. The chest cage gives the lungs a definite shape and supports the lungs from the outside.

The bottom of the chest joins the abdomen, which holds the intestines, the liver, the kidneys and all of the organs which help you digest food and get rid of waste. A large, domed sheet of muscle and fibrous tissue, called the *diaphragm,* separates the lungs from the stomach and the other organs in the abdomen.

When you relax and take a deep breath, you can feel your chest expand, your belly pooch out, cool dry air flows into your nose or mouth. The diaphragm attaches around its edge to the lower back and rib cage. Because of its dome shape, when it contracts, that dome flattens out and moves downward, pulling the bottoms of the lungs with it. At the same time, the *intercostal muscles* between the ribs pull to lift the rib cage up and out, and when you work hard, some neck muscles help. The lung opens in all directions and like a bellows, pulls air in and down the airways into the airs sacs. As air is being pulled in, the airways are wide open, pulled to their widest by the opening of the lung.

Figure 6   Lung volume in healthy and emphysemic lungs

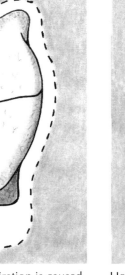

In the healthy person, inspiration is caused by the bellows-like action of the diaphragm and the muscles of the rib cage and neck as they expand the lung, followed by expiration as the structures relax. The chest and lungs deflate like a balloon. The change in size of the lungs (shown as white space) determines the volume of air in each breath.

However, in the person with emphysema, the lung is enlarged but stiff and inflexible, so the volume of air in each breath is much reduced.

When you let air out, all the muscles that have been pulling open relax, let go, and everything springs back to its usual place, the airways becoming narrower as the air is forced out. For a healthy person all it takes to get the air out is this automatic springing back.

When you develop emphysema, the alveoli are destroyed, the elastic abilities of the lung are lost, and they no longer empty automatically. You have to push the air out to exhale. What was a very easy process is now a lot of work.

The Gases We Breathe

Air is mostly made up of two gases, oxygen and nitrogen. Oxygen is about 21% or one-fifth of the total. Oxygen is absorbed from the air because it is able to pass through the very thin wall of the alveolar sac. After it passes through the wall, most of the oxygen attaches itself to a particle in the blood called *hemoglobin*, but some oxygen floats free in the blood. Hemoglobin carries oxygen much more efficiently than floating it in the blood.

Because of the pumping action of the heart, blood travels through *arteries* which split into smaller divisions called *capillaries*. These capillaries, like the ones in the lung around the alveolar sacs, are very close to the individual cells of different tissues. Oxygen is moved by the blood through capillaries to where it can be used in muscle cells, brain cells, etc. Carbon dioxide is a waste product and must be gotten rid of in just the right amounts. It is important in keeping the chemical balance of our bodies. Getting rid of too much can cause problems. Capillaries transfer blood from the alveoli of the lungs to vessels carrying blood into the heart. Capillaries also transfer blood from other body tissues to *veins* carrying

Figure 7   Oxygen and carbon dioxide pass between the air and the blood

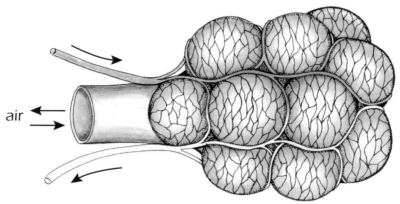

Healthy, normal air sacs (alveoli) are covered with a dense network of tiny blood vessels (capillaries or arterioles) that bring blood into direct contact with the surface of each alveolus.

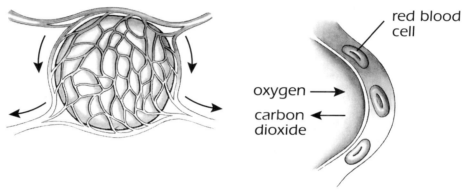

A healthy, normal air sac (alveolus) is covered with a dense network of tiny blood vessels (capillaries or arterioles) close to the air inside the alveolus.

Oxygen passes from the alveolus into the blood where it is captured by the red blood cells, and carbon dioxide is released out of the blood cell into the alveolus.

blood back to the heart. We have two almost separate systems of arteries/capillaries/veins. The left side of the heart receives freshly oxygenated blood from the lungs and sends it to the body. The right side of the heart receives blood from the body and pushes it into the lungs where it releases carbon dioxide and receives oxygen.

When oxygen enters the cells it is used to produce energy, without which the cells would die. In return cells give off carbon dioxide, a waste product which passes back through the capillary wall and into the blood. This carbon-dioxide rich blood is then returned to the lung, back through the walls of the alveolar sacs into the alveoli and bronchi. When you exhale the carbon dioxide leaves your body. Oxygen and carbon dioxide pass through the walls of the air sacs or alveoli, into the blood vessels in the process called *diffusion.*

I've been told by a couple of pulmonologists that my diffusion capacity is severely impaired (out of proportion to the emphysema), functioning at about 25% of predicted capacity.

JVT

The Importance of Oxygen

We need oxygen to stay alive. Oxygen is the major driver of all the body's metabolism, the actions of the body which make proteins, digest food, generate a heart beat, and think.

As your breathing muscles are always working they need a large and constant supply of oxygen. By training the breathing muscles, a small improvement can be made that, while not important for a normal person, can be life-saving for someone with lung disease.

Every process needs oxygen. When we don't have enough oxygen, all activities are slowed or disrupted. An early sign of low oxygen level is that you don't think clearly. As the situation gets worse, the heart begins to fail, doesn't pump blood effectively, and everything just shuts down. In a very few minutes, without oxygen, you die.

In COPD, the loss of oxygen is gradual, occurring over a period of years, unless you have a major illness. Blockage of abnormally-narrowed bronchial tubes, as well as lack of blood vessels around the alveoli, contributes to low oxygen levels. There's plenty of oxygen in the air, it just can't get through the lungs into the blood. When the oxygen in the blood gets low enough, the heart doesn't work as well as usual. We call this problem *cor pulmonale,* from two Latin words meaning heart lungs. The heart still pumps blood, but it doesn't empty as it should with every heart beat. Blood eventually piles up behind the heart, just as water does behind a dam which is only partially open. When this happens, you may develop congestion with fluid accumulating first in your feet, then in other parts of your body.

The Brain: Control Center

Your brain tells your breathing muscles to work by sending signals along your nerves. Your body communicates to the brain that it needs more air in several ways. Lack of oxygen, increased carbon dioxide, putting a stretch on joints or lungs or muscle, pressure on large blood vessels, rise in body temperature and changes in the chemical balance of the body can all be sensed by the special nerves which talk to the breathing centers of the brain. The speed or depth of breathing changes in response to these signals.

The strongest signal to breathe comes from too much carbon dioxide in the blood. But in people with sick lungs, the amount of carbon dioxide in the blood slowly increases over many years so that the brain no longer signals properly. These people depend on other senses to know when they need more air. Lack of oxygen is the most important alternative.

Again the first signals of impending failure occur during exertion. However, most individuals do not recognize these as being abnormal and thus continue smoking until significant damage occurs.   *RC*

How Altitude Affects Breathing

At sea level, the air surrounding us and pushing down on us is at a pressure of one atmosphere, or 760 mm Hg. This is the pressure that can support a column of mercury (Hg) to a height of 760 mm. Weather patterns are associated with small changes in barometric or atmospheric pressure. At a higher altitude air becomes thinner. What this actually means is that the barometric pressure is lower, even though there is the same percent of oxygen in the air. When the pressure is lower, there are fewer particles of air, so that there are fewer particles of oxygen available. This is why with mild or moderate lung disease, you may not be short of breath at sea level when resting but when you are in the mountains or when you fly, you experience increasing difficulty. Therefore, to survive at higher altitude you must breathe extra oxygen.

Mechanisms to Protect the Lung

Your body has several protective mechanisms which help shield the lung from inhaling damaging particles.

The Nose and Upper Airways

As a breath begins, the air moves through the nose and is filtered by the nasal hairs. Some of the foreign particles in the air attach to the sticky mucus in the nose or to the lining. The air is warmed if it is cooler than body temperature and moisture is added. Particles which escape the traps in the nose or the back of the throat may be caught by the mucus which lines the bronchial tubes. This mucus is kept moving upward by the wave action of the cilia, carrying mucus and particles away from the lungs.

Coughing

A cough, aggravating though it may be, is protective because it dislodges mucus and the particles trapped in the mucus. Coughing occurs if you breathe in any larger particle that irritates the airways or if you choke on food or drink, so that it "goes down the wrong pipe." A cough often (though not always) signals contact with a respiratory irritant and is a warning to avoid the material.

Alveolar Macrophages: Defender Cells

Within the lungs are more protective mechanisms. The lungs have a constant supply of *alveolar macrophages*, which pick up foreign particles or invaders. These cells are like security guards which recognize that something doesn't belong. Most of the time, these cells try to destroy the invader by surrounding it, then using enzymes to dissolve it. These counterattacks with enzymes by the body's defending cells are usually successful and many infections from invading bacteria or viruses are prevented.

Enzymes and Enzyme Blockers

After the invader in the lung is neutralized or destroyed by the enzymes, it is very important for the lung to be able to turn off those enzymes so they don't damage normal tissue. To do this the lungs have a supply of another chemical, a protein called *alpha-1 antitrypsin*, which blocks the excess enzymes. If this protein is in short supply, the enzymes remain in the lung and can do severe damage to the structure of the lung.

Antibodies

The body also makes chemicals called *antibodies*, which attach to invaders and destroy them. Antibodies are more successful against some kinds of invaders than others.

Figure 8   Defender cells destroy foreign bodies

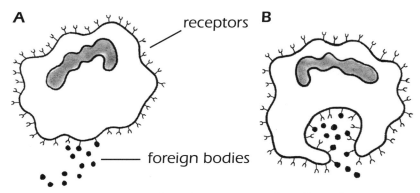

A: Receptors on the surface of the alveolar macrophage cell sense invading foreign bodies.

B: The cell membrane surrounds the foreign bodies and engulfs them.

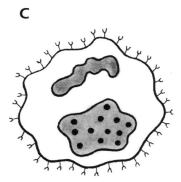

C: Enzymes are released to digest and destroy the foreign bodies. When the cell dies, the enzymes are released into the alveoli or bronchial tubes and may damage the tissue.

Figure 9   Enzymes may attack the lungs and cause emphysema

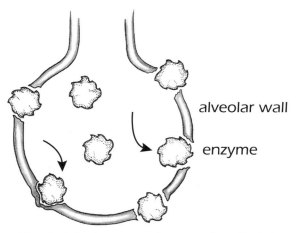

Chemicals in cigarette smoke attract the cells designed to repel invaders to the lungs, where they release enzymes—now known to be primarily responsible for causing emphysema by dissolving or digesting the walls of the alveolar sacs.

Infections

None of the protective systems are perfect. Sometimes they are overwhelmed by huge numbers of invaders and other times, they fail to destroy the invader. When that happens, you can develop a lung infection such as bronchitis or *pneumonia* (an infection of part of the lung).

People who have diseases such as diabetes, or who use medicines such as steroids on a long term basis, may have a greater chance of developing lung infections. These diseases and medications may damage the immune system which provides the defenders and makes the antibodies. Damage makes it more likely that the invader will initiate a full scale infection and overwhelm the defending cells.

Smoking Damage

Smoking damages protective systems. Cigarette smoke is made up of many chemicals, some of which attract the cells designed to repel invaders. When these cells arrive in the lung, even though there is no invader, they may release their packets of enzymes, which are destructive not only to invaders, but to the body's own tissue. Over years of smoking, millions of these defender cells come to the lung and eventually they may damage or destroy large parts of the lung by releasing too much enzyme, and releasing enzymes inappropriately. These enzymes are now known to be primarily responsible for causing emphysema by dissolving the walls of the alveolar sacs. This is why cutting down on the number of cigarettes smoked each day usually doesn't make a big improvement in breathing. Even a very few cigarettes smoked each day can continue to attract defender cells with their damaging enzymes.

Chemicals in smoke may be responsible for keeping the bronchial tubes irritated. With irritation the bronchi produce too much mucus. There may also be spasm or cramping of the muscle around the bronchial tubes causing them to narrow and making breathing more difficult. This leads to chronic bronchitis or asthmatic bronchitis.

Inherited Form of Emphysema

In one type of emphysema that is inherited, the lung's ability to turn off enzymes is severely limited because the protein which normally does this is in short supply. We call this disease *alpha-1 antitrypsin deficiency emphysema*. This is a cause of emphysema unrelated to smoking.

Shortness of Breath (Dyspnea)

Shortness of breath or *dyspnea* is the most-reported complaint for people with COPD. Dyspnea is insidious in its onset, usually occurring only after significant lung injury. It occurs first when COPD has only damaged a small amount of the lung, as difficulty breathing during exertion. It may be dismissed as a result of working too hard or getting older. However, as the disease advances, eventually, dyspnea may be present during the simplest of efforts and at rest. This is very advanced disease. Sudden worsening of dyspnea may be experienced with acute bouts of infection, or with bronchospasm.

Figure 10   Interior of healthy and emphysemic alveoli

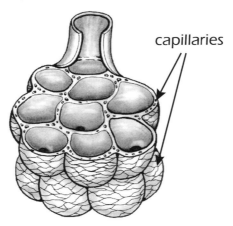
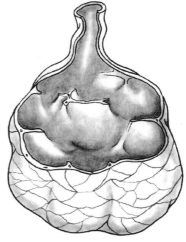

capillaries

The healthy network of capillaries (tiny blood vessels) envelops each air sac (alveolus). The interior walls (seen in cutaway view) provide a large area of surface contact between the blood vessels and the air chambers.

With emphysema, a typical alveolar sac shows the loss of the inner walls. The remaining structure has very little flexibility, there are no inner networks of blood vessels, and the remaining blood vessels provide a much smaller surface area for exchange between blood and air. Oxygen can't get into the blood and the carbon dioxide can't get out.

A number of measures can help reduce shortness of breath:

- Use long-acting bronchodilators such as salmeterol or formoterol. See *Medications for COPD* on page 69.
- If you have been prescribed a quick-acting bronchodilator, use it 20 minutes before activity. See *Medications for COPD* on page 69.
- Use pursed-lips breathing to reduce dyspnea and increase oxygenation. See *Pursed-lip Breathing* on page 45.
- Use diaphragmatic breathing for control. Practice it for thirty minutes to an hour per day to improve respiratory-muscle strength, decrease respiratory rates, and increase the depth or tidal volume of breathing. See *Diaphragmatic Breathing* on page 47.

WARNING: **If you have a sudden increase in dyspnea which cannot be explained by your activity, talk with your doctor. Dyspnea is also a primary complaint for people with other disease, such as heart, kidney, and blood diseases.**

Techniques to Control Dyspnea and Anxiety

Feeling Helpless

According to Gary Paluba, Ph.D., a psychologist who helps people deal with stress, the way to avoid depression and anxiety is to identify the source of the fear and helplessness, and obtain the tools to enable you to gain control. When you feel breathless, experience dyspnea (are short of breath) or can't breathe, you may feel closed in and helpless. You can have a panic or anxiety attack because you fear losing control. Dr. Paluba explains that pursed lip breathing and diaphragmatic breathing are excellent tools for being in control. Pursed lip breathing helps gain control over shortness of breath. Diaphragmatic breathing is very helpful in producing feelings of calm and relaxation.

Anxiety

You feel fear when faced with an actual, immediate threat or emergency; your body prepares for 'fight or flight.' Your heart beats faster and many other physical and emotional changes take place in your body. Likewise, when you anticipate being helpless and powerless, you become extremely alert as if actually facing an emergency. Waiting for the emergency to happen is what psychologists call anxiety: a condition of feeling powerless and helpless in the face of something which has not yet happened. These feelings can also lead to depression.

When you are anxious your body needs even more oxygen than usual but your breathing tends to get shallow, using just the chest to breathe. Your shallow breathing is less efficient so you get less oxygen just when your body needs more. The lack of oxygen and the extra effort you are making to breathe combine to make you feel you have lost control, and you may have a panic or anxiety attack.

How breathing techniques control and prevent anxiety

Diaphragmatic breathing can reverse this process by making your breathing more effective, giving your body more oxygen, helping to slow your heart to your normal rate, and helping you to feel in control and relaxed. Pursed lip breathing helps overcome shortness of breath.

Pursed lip breathing and diaphragmatic breathing are two excellent tools that help you to feel in control and empowered to deal with problems affecting your breathing.

Talk with your doctor about using these techniques and ask your doctor for advice and help for unusual breathing problems or feelings of helplessness.

Practice these techniques and you will be able to take control of your breathing and anxiety, and you will feel calm and relaxed and better able to cope.   *JVT*

Don't Panic: Sudden Shortness of Breath

Even a mild change in breathing conditions can be frightening for people with lung disease. The important thing to remember is, don't panic! If breathing becomes more difficult, sit and lean forward slightly. Pursed-lip breathing usually helps, and relaxation techniques. Inhale from a bronchodilator aerosol like albuterol with or without atrovent as soon as shortness of breath gets going. It will do no harm and is likely to reverse the attack. It is wise to learn to deal with such episodes, and to be able to determine the difference between a mild change (which is mostly controllable), and a sudden, severe change, a real emergency.

Sudden and/or severe chest pains or shortness of breath are the most common emergencies in COPD. Before calling your doctor in what you perceive to be an emergency, ask yourself if you have:

- A noticeable change in your symptoms, particularly if this change lasts more than one day

- Any new symptoms.

Learn to differentiate between good days, bad days, and emergencies. Some changes or symptoms that might be important are:

- Unusually increased shortness of breath, added difficulty in breathing, or increased wheezing
- Increased coughing, more frequent, more severe, or both
- Increased sputum production
- Change in color of sputum to yellow, grey or green
- Change in consistency of sputum, thicker, stickier
- Fever
- Swelling ankles, legs, or around eyes
- Sudden weight gain of three to five pounds overnight
- Palpitations of the heart or pulse faster than usual
- Unusual dizziness, sleepiness, headaches, visual disturbances, irritability, or trouble thinking
- Unusual loss of appetite
- Dehydration, evidenced by concentrated urine and dryness of skin
- Chest pains
- Blood in sputum, urine, or bowel movement.

Emergencies

Plan while you are thinking clearly, so that you know what to do in case of an emergency. The first step should be to contact your doctor. But emergencies often develop during your doctor's off-time. If the situation is serious, dial 911, and state the emergency facility you should be taken to. Have a written plan that you keep close by the telephone, or inside the cover of the directory with your doctor's number, and the name and phone number of your nearest relative. If you are frightened and in a state of panic, you may not be able to remember phone numbers. The paramedics will place a call for you to your relative, if you have the number nearby. They are usually trained to look beside the phone and on the refrigerator door for critical information.

The American Lung Association provides cards that you can fill out with personal information, medical history, name and number of your doctor, next of kin, medications, conditions, and allergies. Send for one, fill it out, and keep it on your refrigerator door with a fridge magnet. Paramedics can be pointed to it, even if you are having trouble talking.

Our local Police Departments on the Cape will provide "File of Life" folders (See *Symptoms Checklist* on page 217) for the same purpose, enclosed in a magnet to attach to refrigerator doors.   *JVT*

Aspects of Breathing We Can Control

With COPD you can't take breathing for granted. You need to draw in more air and use it more effectively than before. You also need to learn to avoid bad breathing habits, learn to control your breathing.

Depth of the breath: some people breathe with only the upper part of their chest, and don't use the diaphragm. This means that air doesn't get down into the lower lobes of the lungs where most of the gas exchange takes place. Learn to make better use of your diaphragm.

Pace of breath: you can also control how fast you breathe. When you take short shallow pants, you inhale and exhale so fast that new, oxygenated air doesn't get to the lower lobes of the lungs.

Tension in respiratory muscles: sometimes, due to physical or psychological tension, you hold your shoulders very tight. The abdominal muscles might also tighten up making it harder to breathe. You can relax these muscles by breathing deeply and evenly in a more relaxed fashion.

Techniques for breathing are given in the following pages.

Rules for Better Breathing

Illness can affect your breathing system in many ways, but educating yourself about COPD will help you to understand how it happens, and possibly prevent problems. *You* are the most important part of the breathing system. Use good sense to protect yourself. Here is a short list of rules for better breathing. Learn to pay attention to the signals from your body, and apply these rules to protect your body and to preserve your quality of life.

- Avoid harm. Be aware of things around you which harm your lungs: cigarettes, second-hand smoke, job-related exposures, air pollution, perfumes.
- Take good care of yourself. Don't smoke. Eat sensibly, get regular exercise.
- Don't be manipulated into physical exertion that is too stressful. Respect your body, and demand the same kind of respect from others.
- Do exercise regularly. This improves overall body efficiency and helps control dyspnea.
- Get plenty of rest. A run-down, tired body has very little resistance to infections.
- Don't subject yourself to viruses and germs, when the situation can be avoided. Your grandchildren's colds can be the worst culprits!
- Be frank with your family and friends about it. Don't suffer silently, knowing that a contagious illness is being coughed or sneezed upon you.
- Wash your hands frequently with anti-bacterial soap.
- Use correctly the tools you have for breathing: diaphragm, chest muscles, posture, relaxation, etc.
- Keep your nebulizers clean and maintain your oxygen equipment.

Tools for Better Breathing

Pursed-lip Breathing

Pursed-lips simply means that your lips are in a whistle or puckered or kissing position. Pursed-lips breathing helps you relieve shortness of breath. The resistance created by breathing out through semi-closed lips creates a slight back pressure in the lungs, which may act to keep damaged airways open instead of collapsing and creating airway obstruction. This controlled breathing exhales more used air and inhales more clean air, increasing the amount of oxygen delivered to the lungs and blood. Pursed-lips breathing slows the breathing pattern for more efficiency. This technique is important in short-of-breath panic when breathing becomes rapid and shallow, with increasing shortness of breath.

The technique of pursed-lips breathing is simple but must be practiced daily for the greatest benefit. Use pursed-lips breathing whenever you feel short of breath, to reinforce its use during more-than-average shortness of breath. If shortness of breath is increasing and there is no apparent reason, contact your doctor and find the cause.

Figure 11   Pursed-lips breathing

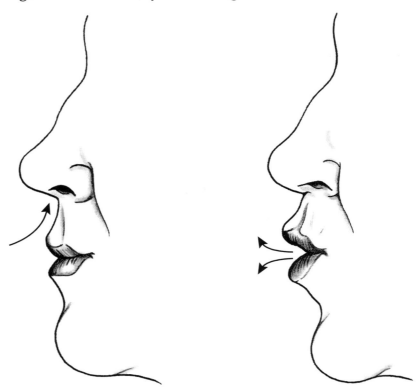

Pursed-lips breathing helps you relieve shortness of breath. A: Inhale normally through your nose with your mouth closed.

B: Position your lips in a pursed or kissing position and exhale with modest resistance until almost all the stale air in your lungs is pushed out. Exhale slowly, taking twice as long to exhale as you do to inhale.

How to breathe with pursed lips

1 Inhale normally through your nose with your mouth closed.

2 Position your lips in a pursed or kissing position and exhale with modest resistance until almost all the stale air in your lungs is pushed out. You should hear the air moving past your lips.

3 Take twice as long to exhale as to inhale. Practice by counting or tapping to a rhythm. For example, breathe in for two seconds while counting (one thousand and one, one thousand and two) and breathe out for four or five counts.

4 Continue pursed-lips breathing until you have completely recovered.

Practice pursed-lips breathing whenever you exert yourself and feel short of breath. For example, practice while climbing stairs.

Diaphragmatic Breathing

Diaphragmatic breathing is another technique to control shortness of breath. Like the other techniques it must be practiced and used daily. Use the technique daily in combination with pursed-lips breathing or whenever you become short-of-breath.

Diaphragmatic breathing strengthens the diaphragm—the primary breathing muscle. Normally the diaphragm does about 80% of the work of breathing, is rounded and the rib cage is in a normal position. With COPD, the diaphragm muscle becomes flat, less able to perform normally, and the rib cage expands. As this change occurs the accessory muscles of the chest do more work. This process is inefficient, more oxygen is needed to power the other muscles for breathing, and shortness-of-breath increases. Diaphragmatic breathing can help reduce shortness-of-breath.

Learning to breathe with the diaphragm

1 Get comfortable, either seated in a chair or lying on your back on a comfortable surface.

2 Place one hand in the center of your stomach at the base of the breastbone, then sniff. You should be able to feel the movement of the diaphragm when you sniff. Or, lie on your back and place a book on your belly button; it will move when your stomach rises due to the movement of the diaphragm.

3 Place your other hand on your upper chest to detect changes in position and activity of the chest muscles.

4 Exhale slowly through pursed lips while pulling your abdominal muscles tight—inward and squeezing upward. Then inhale slowly through your nose. Your abdomen should expand downward and outward. You should feel the most movement in the hand on your stomach.

5 Concentrate on breathing slowly and deeply, twice as long for exhaling as for inhaling. Concentrate on keeping your chest as still as possible and focus all movement in your abdomen. This will refocus movement to the diaphragm muscle where it should be.

6 After several trials, relax. If you feel that you are becoming light-headed, slow your breathing and relax for a short time.

You may need to practice inhaling very slowly in order to make the diaphragm work. If you feel light-headed or need to inhale after exhaling for only two counts, you may not be doing diaphragmatic breathing.

After you have mastered diaphragmatic breathing, you can use it for relaxation or to reduce anxiety any time. You can do it anywhere, sitting down, standing up, or lying down. You can take 10, 15, or more diaphragmatic breaths as often as you want. Concentrate on making the inhalations as long as possible, for a count of four or five. Your exhalations will be about equal in length.

To strengthen and redirect muscle activation to your diaphragm, practice the technique daily.

Figure 12   Diaphragmatic breathing

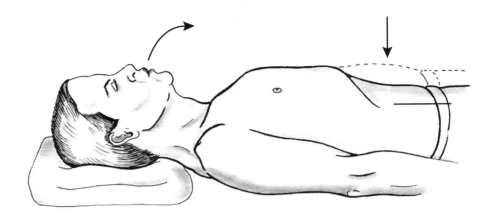

Diaphragmatic breathing is very helpful in producing feelings of calm and relaxation as well as to control shortness of breath. Exhale slowly through pursed lips while pulling your abdominal muscles tight—inward and squeezing upward.

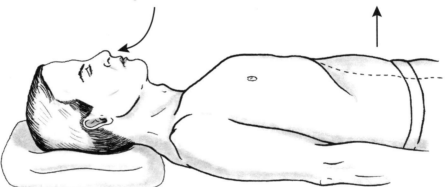

Then inhale slowly through your nose. Your abdomen should expand downward and outward. If you place one hand on your chest and the other on your stomach, you should feel more movement on your stomach.

COPD Defined

Pulmonary Diseases

Chronic obstructive pulmonary disease (COPD) and chronic obstructive lung disease (COLD) are terms that the medical profession uses for chronic bronchitis, asthmatic bronchitis, and emphysema. They share a common trait: persistent difficulty in getting the air to flow out of the lung normally. Once these chronic diseases or processes start, you can never be normal again. You may have just one disease, or two, or all three. The three diseases often overlap in one person. For example, as well as emphysema, you may have chronic bronchitis making you cough, with asthmatic bronchitis making you wheeze.

Other obstructive lung diseases belong in this group but are quite different in their cause and somewhat different in their treatment. Although they're not the focus of this book, they are *asthma*, *bronchiectasis*, and *inherited emphysema*. Asthma, as it occurs in most lifetime non-smokers, is quite different in that most people with it have normal breathing most of the time. Bronchiectasis, although it is a chronic process, is not caused by cigarette smoke as most COPD is, but by genetic problems such as cystic fibrosis or severe childhood infection. Inherited emphysema is caused by the destruction of alveolar sacs by enzymes in the absence of alpha-1 antitrypsin.

Figure 13   Three types of airway obstruction

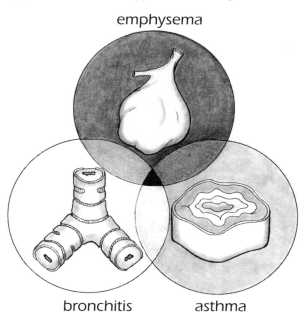

emphysema

bronchitis   asthma

Emphysema, bronchitis, and asthma can be found separately but they often overlap in one person. You may have just one disease, or two, or all three.

Table 1: COPD and other pulmonary diseases

Disease	Symptoms				Description and cause
	Cough	Wheeze	Mucus	Dyspnea[a]	
Emphysema	yes			yes	Destruction or enlargement of alveolar sacs. Often caused by smoking. Causes dyspnea (shortness of breath, "SOB") and may cause coughing.
Chronic Bronchitis	yes	often	yes	yes	Long-term, excessive production of mucus by the trachea and bronchial tubes. Often caused by smoking.
Asthmatic Bronchitis		yes	yes	yes, during attack	Bronchitis associated with wheezing and rapid changes in ability to breathe, similar to asthma. Treatment for asthmatic bronchitis may be different than treating either asthma or bronchitis alone.
Acute Bronchitis	yes	often	yes	yes	The mucous membranes of the bronchial tubes are inflamed by infection, allergy, air-borne materials, cold air.
Asthma	yes	yes		yes, during attack	Extreme allergic reaction resulting in constriction of the bronchial airway. Often the patient is normal between attacks.
Inherited emphysema: alpha-1 antitrypsin deficiency	yes			yes	Emphysema. The destruction of alveolar sacs by enzymes in the absence of alpha-1 antitrypsin. An inherited deficiency, causing emphysema.
Bronchiectasis	yes		large amounts		Chronic dilation of bronchial tubes with secondary infection in lower part of lung. Usually caused by a prior infection.

a. Dyspnea varies with severity of disease and worsens with exacerbations

Chronic Bronchitis

Chronic bronchitis is diagnosed when there is a history of excessive *mucus* production (also called *sputum* or *phlegm*) with cough on most days for three or more months, and recurring yearly for at least two years. Most people with chronic bronchitis cough much more than this, and bring up a lot of mucus almost every day, especially on getting up in the morning.

Cause and symptoms

The most common cause of chronic bronchitis is long exposure to the damaging substances in cigarette smoke. Less common is long exposure to air pollution, and breathing in dust for a long time. These substances cause the lining of the bronchial tubes to become irritated or inflamed. Then the mucus glands in the airways produce more and thicker sputum. The delicate cilia, the tiny hair-like structures in the bronchial tubes responsible for the upward movement of mucus, become damaged, can no longer work in cooperation, and are not effective in clearing mucus out of the lungs. Excess mucus stays longer in the bronchial tubes and makes the airways, which are normally sterile and free of bacteria, more susceptible to infection.

Chronic bronchitis begins slowly as sputum production increases, due to more cells making mucus, and enlargement of the mucus glands. A morning cough may develop. In winter, or anytime you have a cold or an upper respiratory infection, longer periods of sputum production may occur. This process continues until mucus secretion is continuous. At some point, the airways swell, making them narrower and causing the bronchial tube muscles to spasm. With narrowing of the bronchial tubes, muscle spasm, and partial filling of the tubes with mucus, it becomes harder to breathe. Then wheezing may begin, and you may be diagnosed with asthmatic bronchitis.

At first, your difficulty in breathing is with increased activity. However, in time, you may become short of breath even in normal activities. As a result, you tend to do less and less to avoid shortness of breath.

As your disease gets worse other problems may occur. Oxygen level in the blood may fall as your airway becomes plugged by phlegm. If the low oxygen level is not corrected, it can lead to problems with thinking. You become more and more anxious, even depressed. You may become upset or hostile because it seems no one is helping you.

Also as a result of low oxygen level, increased strain is placed on your heart, so that it doesn't pump as well as it should. Medically, this is heart failure. When this occurs, you notice your feet swelling and possibly your abdomen. Extra oxygen may bring you relief, but eventually, even with extra oxygen, your lungs fail to keep up with your need to breathe and you die.

Prevention and control

Chronic bronchitis is associated with long exposure to cigarette smoke, usually for more than 20 years, and usually because you yourself smoke. It may also occur because you are exposed to second-hand smoke, that is, someone else's smoking. Second-hand smoke seems to be most dangerous when you live with a smoker.

Some people who smoke, even heavily, never develop chronic bronchitis. Doctors do not completely understand why some develop lung disease and others don't. We know some factors, but we cannot always predict who will develop lung problems. You can inherit a tendency toward lung disease, being more likely to get it if family members are bronchitic. Exposure to cigarette smoke in infancy or young childhood also makes you more likely to develop chronic bronchitis and other infections of the breathing system, which may result in development of lung disease as an adult. We know that once the bronchitic process starts, it doesn't stop, and that it accelerates with continued exposure to damaging substances. That is, the disease will get worse faster if you continue to smoke or work around dusts and air pollution than if you avoid exposure. So, if you have been diagnosed with chronic bronchitis, avoid contact with irritating fumes or dusts.

With chronic bronchitis, especially with asthmatic bronchitis, you may also have allergy symptoms such as: runny nose, sinus problems, postnasal drip and wheezing after exposure to house dust, molds, certain blooming or seeding plants, or animals such as cats. If you have these symptoms, you need to protect yourself, and you may also need anti-allergy treatment.

Until quite recently, we thought that nothing could be done to prevent bronchitis from getting worse, except to avoid breathing in damaging materials. Now there are medications which can slow the progress of bronchitis, as well as improve symptoms, so you can lead a more normal life. These medications include inhaled drugs which slow down or stop the inflammation that continues bronchial-tube damage. These medications are discussed in more detail in *Medications for COPD* on page 69.

Emphysema

Pulmonary emphysema is quite different from chronic bronchitis, although both types of lung damage often co-exist. Emphysema is destruction of the structure of the lung. In bronchitis, the bronchial tubes are still there, even though they are not normal. In emphysema, large numbers of alveolar sacs are destroyed in parts of the lung. The remaining alveolar sacs become enlarged, and do not function normally. They no longer have the normal number of capillaries next to them, essential for transfer of oxygen from the air in the alveoli to the blood. So even though you keep breathing in and out of these damaged areas, oxygen is unable to transfer efficiently to the blood.

Alveolar destruction also results in a loss of the elastic nature of the lung. Normally, the lung is able to be blown up, then shrink and expel air easily, because of the elastic qualities of the alveolar sacs. As these are destroyed, the lung can no longer expel air easily. Besides this, the elastic alveolar sacs also help to hold the tiniest bronchial tubes open by pulling on them. When the alveolar sacs are destroyed, the airways begin to collapse. These changes are irreversible, they never go away. You can never grow new alveolar sacs. However, you can make the remaining alveolar sacs as efficient as possible.

Cause and symptoms

Emphysema has many causes, but the most common is cigarette smoking. Certain chemicals in cigarette smoke attract cells to the lung. These cells release damaging enzymes, which destroy lung tissue. Historically, men were affected with emphysema more than women, probably because men were more likely to be smokers. However, as women are smoking more today, there is an increase in the number of women with emphysema. More than 90% of people with emphysema in various studies were heavy smokers, typically consuming more than one pack of cigarettes per day for many years. One pack per day equals twenty cigarettes per day. For one year this is called a *one pack-year* consumption history. Twenty cigarettes or one pack per day for ten years, is a *ten pack-year* history. Most people with emphysema due to cigarette smoking have at least a 20 pack-year history before symptoms become bad enough to seek medical assistance.

Figure 14   Comparison of healthy with diseased airways

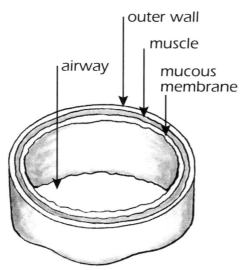

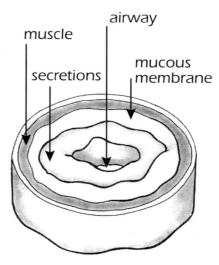

The normal airway is formed by the outer wall, muscle, and mucous membrane, with a large open air passage.

In bronchitis, the mucous membrane is swollen, the muscle is inflamed, and excessive secretions all combine to reduce the size of the air passage.

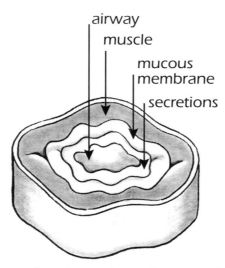

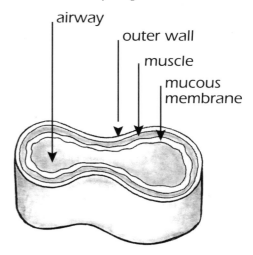

In asthma, the muscle goes into spasm, the mucous membrane is swollen, and excessive secretions all combine to narrow the airway.

In emphysema, the muscle is inflamed, the airway is flabby and compressed, but the airway passage is still open.

Emphysema can be an inherited disease. A lack of the protein *alpha-1 antitrypsin* is the cause. This protein blocks the effects of some enzymes, and stops infection or chemical damage which in turn stops damage to the lungs. The good news is that a replacement alpha-1 antitrypsin drug is available. The bad news is that the cost can exceed $50,000 per year.

Occupational exposure to cadmium and possibly to other substances present in some industries can also result in emphysema.

Emphysema begins slowly but is progressive, that is, it gets worse. The first symptom most people notice is shortness of breath or dyspnea during activity, and shortness-of-breath on rising in the morning. As emphysema gets worse, shortness of breath is present even at rest. This shortness-of-breath can be relieved by resting and sometimes by lying down or sitting leaning forward.

Coughing, usually dry, so that no sputum is coughed up, is also a common complaint. But as emphysema is associated with chronic bronchitis, coughing may bring up mucus.

As emphysema gets worse, the heart has to work harder and harder, and may begin to fail causing congestive heart failure or cor pulmonale. If you have emphysema badly enough to cause cor pulmonale, your life expectancy can be quite limited. But usually emphysema relates to difficulty breathing more than any other symptom.

Prevention and control

Whether or not a person has symptoms depends on how extensive the emphysema is and how much normal lung tissue is left to do the work of breathing. Certainly if you have COPD, you and everyone in your family should all avoid smoking, as you are at higher risk of developing symptomatic emphysema.

If emphysema is severe, a lung transplant is an option in some cases.

The treatment for each component of COPD—emphysema and chronic bronchitis—is essentially the same regardless of the cause of the disease component. The symptoms of shortness of breath, cough, sputum production, and wheezing are treated with the same medications and procedures in all patients with those symptoms. Thus, emphysema is treated in essentially the same way if it has been caused by cigarette smoking or by the effects of the inherited deficiency of the alpha-1 antitrypsin enzyme. In addition, the smoker needs to stop smoking; the person with the inherited deficiency may benefit from replacement therapy.

Inherited emphysema

Although it is possible to replace alpha-1 antitrypsin by regular injection, it has not yet been proven that giving the protein in this way will prevent further emphysema from developing. If you are diagnosed with emphysema before age 50, or have emphysema and never smoked, or have relatives with emphysema, get your doctor to check how much alpha-1 antitrypsin you have in your blood. If the level is low, you can consider replacement therapy. Also consider testing children and other relatives.

The outlook for prevention of inherited emphysema as a result of a lack of alpha-1 antitrypsin is more hopeful now than in the past. Several pharmaceuticals are available or being prepared for market. Several clinical trials of new treatments are in progress; the Alpha One Foundation is a good source for information.

The Progress of COPD

COPD is a progressive disease, but does not get steadily worse in most people. Progression can be slowed. Studies of large groups of people with COPD show that they fall into two groups: those who still smoke and those who don't. Those who continue to smoke are much more likely to have steadily weakening lungs, so that all the symptoms, particularly shortness of breath and cough, become increasingly severe. These people are more likely to die of COPD. The continuing smoker with COPD is also at increased risk for lung cancer, compared to the ex-smoker and the smoker who doesn't have COPD.

For the ex-smoker with COPD, the progression of lung disease is less predictable. People with chronic bronchitis who stop smoking may have a significant improvement since they usually will have much less cough and sputum production after they quit. Many ex-smokers do not have much change in their lung function for many years. However, many ex-smokers with COPD become steadily more short of breath and are likely to eventually die because of their COPD. Those who no longer smoke but are still exposed to second hand smoke over several years will probably do worse than ex-smokers who are not exposed to smoke. This is not proven, but is an area where more study is needed. Certainly some ex-smokers are very bothered by inhaling secondhand cigarette smoke and develop immediate shortness of breath.

When Your Breathing Gets Worse

For some reason, people with COPD have a very up-and-down course of disease. One day you may feel great and breathe well, the next day you may be in awful shape. We do not understand why this happens. Many have theories about it. They say that the humidity is higher or lower, that the temperature is too hot or too cold, that something must be in the air. Sometimes they relate increased problems to a family dispute or emotional upset. It is certainly possible that a change in the atmosphere can change COPD for better or worse. Many things not under human control, which people blame, such as weather factors, are hard to avoid.

COPD is a variable process. Changes in barometric pressure and humidity levels can have a significant impact on people with COPD. You may, at times, feel like "walking/talking barometers." The important thing is that things will generally get better again, often by the next day, if you just hang on.

However, sometimes breathing problems do not get better over several days. Along with increased shortness of breath you have increased cough. Sometimes you have a lot of wheezing. Other times, you cough up more than the usual amount of mucus and the mucus turns yellow or green. When symptoms become exaggerated like this, you have an *exacerbation* of your COPD, a worsening, and increase in symptoms.

Why do exacerbations occur? We know some of the causes, but not all.

- Often, the exacerbation is preceded by an upper respiratory infection or a bout of *sinusitis*.
- The exacerbation may occur because of a change, particularly a decrease, in the amount or type of medicine you take. Some medicines even cause bronchospasm and should be avoided. A common example is the group of heart and blood pressure medications called *beta blockers*. Such *beta blockers* are very different from the *beta agonists* used for the treatment of COPD. Always ask your pharmacist if any new medicine might worsen your COPD.
- The exacerbation may follow exposure to an allergic substance or an irritating dust, or to secondhand cigarette smoke.
- Exacerbations are usually due either to increased irritation or inflammation of the bronchial tubes, or to increased narrowing causing wheezing.

Most exacerbations are self-limited. They will get better whether or not they are treated. If you feel the exacerbation is really bad, call for help. Treatment often makes you feel better quicker, and may prevent more severe results, such as the need for hospitalization. Your doctor may change your medications, based on the type of exacerbation you have.

Exacerbation of COPD is usually what brings you to medical attention. *Respiratory failure* can occur, where breathing is so abnormal that you can't get enough oxygen into your blood, and can't get rid of carbon dioxide. Until breathing gets really hard, some people are not willing to go to a doctor, but treating these episodes early can prevent major deterioration of lung function.

Diagnosis of COPD

Diagnosis of the different forms of COPD is usually straight forward and does not require invasive testing. A good history and physical examination is essential. The characteristic history shows gradual onset of shortness of breath, often with cough, phlegm production, or intermittent wheezing. When these symptoms are connected to a history of cigarette smoking and no other obvious cause, the odds are you have COPD. Occasionally, a family history may suggest the possibility of inherited disease.

Physical examination will show abnormal breathing sounds with a long slow exhalation phase, since people with COPD have trouble getting air out. Wheezing may be present. Sometimes crackling sounds can be heard, particularly at the bottoms of the lungs. In severe cases of COPD, weight and muscle loss may be evident. Swelling of the feet may suggest that the heart is not functioning well, and blue fingernails can indicate low oxygen level. With the suspicion of COPD the following tests are often ordered to decide if the diagnosis is correct and to determine how severe the problem is:

- Chest x-ray
- Breathing tests
- Arterial blood gas
- Electrocardiogram
- Exercise testing with oximetry to check oxygen level

Chest X-ray

A common test is the chest x-ray, with two different views of the chest usually made, one from back to front, and one from the side. These two views allow the doctor to see both lungs and to see if the heart looks normal. COPD will show up as larger-than-normal lungs, sometimes with an abnormal position of the diaphragm. The lungs may also look darker than usual due to the destruction of alveolar sacs. Sometimes there are increased markings or lines made by the swollen and damaged bronchial tubes.

If other diseases are present, they will show up as well, for example:

- Lung tumors
- Scar tissue in the lungs from exposure to substances like asbestos, or unexpected infections
- An abnormally large heart shadow suggesting heart disease.

The x-ray does not usually show how bad the disease is, but can indicate another disease which may need further evaluation.

Figure 15   X-ray view of healthy and emphysemic lungs

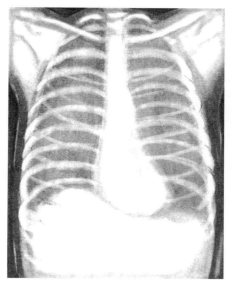 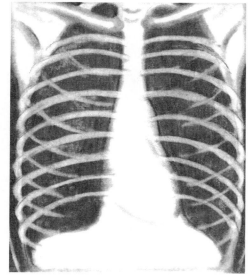

The x-ray allows the doctor to see both lungs and to see if the heart looks normal, with healthy lungs and a dome-shaped diaphragm,

COPD will show up as larger-than-normal lungs, with an abnormal position of the diaphragm. The enlarged lungs have lost flexibility, compressing the diaphragm, and making it difficult to breathe

Breathing Tests

Breathing tests are routinely performed to measure the amount of air you can move out of your lungs in a given time.

Spirometry

The most useful test is *spirometry*, which is done by filling your lungs with air, then blowing out as hard and as fast as you can. This test usually requires all the effort you can muster, as without great effort, the test is useless. See "Spirometry testing" on page 58.

Because effort is so important, the technician often encourages by yelling, "Blast it out! Push harder! Keep pushing, it's still coming out!" Don't get upset. The technician is simply coaching you to do your best. If you are slow to get the air out, you may be requested to take an inhaled medication to enlarge your bronchial tubes. Testing is repeated after 20 to 45 minutes. If the amount of air improves after medication, you may have some *reversibility*, that is, you may respond well to inhaled medications. Testing may also be repeated after other treatment, such as steroids or surgery.

The numerical results from your spirometry test are compared to normal data from thousands of healthy non-smoking people of your age, sex, race, and size. Your numbers are graded as a percent of normal. Sometimes your numbers are graded according to how much they deviate or are different from normal values. If you have performed a spirometry test before, a comparison can be made with your own data. This can show whether you are better or worse, or holding your own.

Figure 16   Spirometry testing

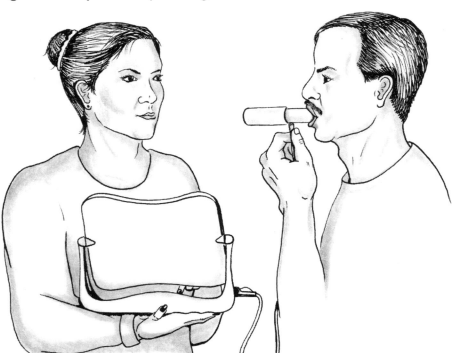

Spirometry is one of the most important breathing tests.

Spirometry does not give all the information necessary to determine whether you have emphysema or bronchitis, or whether you have asthmatic bronchitis. To determine which of these obstructive processes is present, other lung-function tests may be needed.

FEV_1

The most important measurement made during the spirometry, and the one which most doctors mean when they say you have "60% of your lung function," or "half of your lung function" is the amount of air which you can forcibly blow out in one second. This is called FEV_1 (pronounced *eff ee vee one*). FEV_1 is the number which is best at predicting how a person with COPD will do. It helps your doctor decide how much risk there is for a surgical procedure and when to start watching for a low oxygen level in your blood. It can also tell your doctor whether you are likely to die from your lung disease, or from something else. FEV_1 is the main number looked at after you breathe in a medication in the laboratory to see if the medication is likely to help you.

The most common way to measure lung function is the FEV_1 test. When the FEV_1 is less than normal but greater than 60% of the expected value for your age, race, sex, and size (each of these factors has been found to influence these tests), you have mild disease. If the FEV_1 is between 40 and 60% of expected, your disease is moderate. For an FEV_1 less than 40% of expected, disease is severe. The FEV_1 should be measured when you are in your usual state of health, not when you are ill or having increased difficulty. It should be measured after you have used your bronchodilator inhaler, in order to get a true picture of your best value.

Table 2: Use the FEV_1 to determine the severity of your COPD

If your FEV_1 value is:	COPD severity	My COPD severity is:
More than 60% of the normal value for your age, sex, and size	Mild	
Between 40% and 60% of the normal value for your age, sex, and size	Moderate	
Less than 40% of the normal value for your age, sex, and size	Severe	

Peak flow rate testing

Another measure of lung function is the fastest rate at which you can get air out, or *peak flow rate*. Although this test is helpful in asthma, it is not as useful in COPD. The total amount of air which you can get out is also less useful in assessing your illness than the FEV_1. Other lung function tests may help in deciding more about your disease.

Use of a peak flow meter may be helpful in determining whether or not to attempt certain activities. If the peak flow is less than "normal" for you, it can confirm a "bad day." Strenuous physical activity may have to be postponed for a better breathing day.   *JVT*

Arterial Blood Gas and Oximetry Testing

Measuring the oxygen in your blood at rest or during exercise is the best method available to determine if you need extra oxygen either all the time or just during exercise. Normal expected values for oxygen saturation vary depending on altitude, but should be at least 90%. Values less than 90% indicate low oxygen in arterial blood. You may have normal arterial oxygen at rest but lower during exercise. Most exercise specialists feel that a low oxygen level during exercise should be corrected.

Adjustment to the resting oxygen prescription will need to be made. People do *desaturate* (lose blood oxygen) during activity and it is appropriate to compensate by increasing oxygen flow. However, this should only be done under the supervision of a physician.

Arterial blood gas levels are important cues to the severity of and need for treatment of abnormality in your lungs. At some time during the course of COPD, your arterial blood gases will be tested. You will have a small needle inserted in an artery in your wrist to test arterial blood for oxygen and carbon dioxide levels. This test has to be done on arterial blood, that is, blood coming out of your heart, before it circulates to tissues. Blood from a vein will not work, as it has already given up its oxygen to the tissues, and received carbon-dioxide. (You may need two tests, both at the elbow and at the wrist, in order to get all necessary information.)

This test can be painful as the artery is right beside a nerve in the wrist. A local anesthetic such as *lidocaine* is very helpful. Ask the technician to use it, or another anesthetic.

Don't be afraid to ask for the local anesthesia. Also, see tips for visualizing during the procedure, a focus technique that will help the patient to bear these necessary tests, in *Alternatives and Supplements to Medicine* on page 80.

Most people undergoing blood gas studies for the first few times will not have been made aware that the arterial puncture can be less painful with a little local anesthesia. The first nine times blood gases were drawn from me, no local anesthesia was used or offered. I became terrified of going through this procedure, until one technician suggested using a small injection of lidocaine to numb the area of my wrist. While the puncture is still an unpleasant experience, it is less painful.   *JVT*

Arterial blood gas helps your doctor to decide if you need an extra supply of oxygen to get your oxygen level back to normal. After initial measurement of your blood gases, your oxygen level may be rechecked by measuring only the amount of oxygen attached to your hemoglobin. This test is called *oximetry*.

Oximetry is performed with a clothespin-like gadget attached to your finger or ear. Since it is not uncomfortable, this is the test most often repeated on visits to your doctor, and in a hospital. Since your lungs have to work harder when you exercise, this test may be done while you walk or bicycle, to see if you need oxygen during more strenuous activity. The same test may also be done at night, to see if you need overnight oxygen because you sleep poorly and awaken tired, or because you fall asleep during the day.

Arterial blood gas testing also demonstrates how well your lungs are working to get rid of carbon dioxide. Knowing carbon dioxide level helps in evaluating both how well your lungs are working, and whether or not your brain is directing your lungs normally. The carbon dioxide level is an indicator of risk for surgery which needs you to be asleep. Carbon dioxide level also helps to determine how rapidly your disease is progressing, and to some extent, your *prognosis*, or how your future health is going to be affected. Other measurements can also be performed to further evaluate your medical status

Blood Pressure Testing

Blood pressure is measured with a *sphygmomanometer*, or blood-pressure cuff and gauge, and a *stethoscope* to hear the sounds created by pressure in the arteries. Blood pressure is reported as a top and bottom number or *systolic* and *diastolic* pressure. The top or systolic pressure is the number which varies most. The bottom or diastolic pressure remains fairly stable in a normal or disease-free person. Blood pressure is normally written as: 120/80 mm Hg, where 120 is the systolic pressure, 80 is the diastolic pressure, and mm Hg is millimeters of mercury pressure.

As a rule, your systolic pressure should not exceed 140 mm Hg while resting, and your diastolic should be less than 90 to 95 mm Hg.

Miscellaneous Tests

If your lung disease is severe enough to have affected your heart, you may need an *electrocardiogram* (EKG or ECG) or an *echocardiogram*. The EKG will often show cor pulmonale due to lung disease and may be helpful in deciding if you've ever had a heart attack. The echocardiogram tells more about how well your heart works as a pump.

If you want to exercise or if your chief complaint is shortness of breath during exertion the doctor may order an *exercise study*. This study will use a bicycle or a motor-driven treadmill that gradually increases the amount of work you do. You will be closely monitored by ECG, blood pressure, and oximetry; and you may breathe into a mask similar to that used by scuba divers to measure the air you breathe out.

4 Treatment

Medications and Treatments

General Medication Advice

There are many medications for lung disease which may look or taste alike, but which are very different. Know your medications. Know them well, and don't mix them or their means of delivery. This is especially true for inhalers.

Learn the differences between different inhaler medications and their delivery equipment. Mark them differently so you know which are preventative and which are for an immediate problem. The outside cases for inhaler medications are *not* interchangeable—stems on the medication canisters are different, if you swap them, you may not get your medicine. Be careful.

Never take other people's medicines or use their inhalers. Medications prescribed for your wife or friend may be damaging to you, or ineffective. An antibiotic given to a relative for urinary tract infection may not help your bronchitis and may cause a severe allergic reaction.

Many people with COPD are on several medications at once, usually taken at different times, some with a meal, some before or after. Follow your doctor's instructions for the most benefit with the fewest side effects.

To be sure you don't forget to take a medication, there are several possibilities:

- Buy a pillbox from your pharmacy, then place a day's worth of medications in the box.
- Buy a multi-compartment box for several days.
- Put your medications in a place you use a lot, such as a bathroom or kitchen counter.
- Set out your morning medications the night before.

If your medications are changed by your doctor and you start to experience problems, call your doctor or pharmacist immediately.

Be sure to tell all pharmacists and doctors treating you of changes in medications or of changes in your health.

When you visit your doctor's office, bring all your medicines with you.

If you have questions about a medication ask them as soon as possible. Writing a list of questions will help you remember.

A good source of information is a *Physicians' Desk Reference*. Ask your doctor or pharmacist, or at a good library. Other sources of good information regarding medications are available as well. See *Bibliography* on page 233.

Applicators for Medications

Inhalers with spacers, and gas nebulizers are the two types of applicators that deliver medications for COPD. Inhalers are small units that fit in a pocket or a purse, while nebulizers are much larger and work on a different principle. Each type of equipment is used to apply medications by inhaling them. Explanations of each type of equipment follow, with instructions for keeping them clean.

The many different types of inhalers are categorized by their purpose—to prevent or treat bronchospasm,

Metered Dose Inhalers (MDIs) and Spacers

Metered-dose inhalers (MDIs) are also called *puffers,* and are usually activated by pushing down on the canister. They are set to deliver an exact amount of medicine.

It is important to coordinate your breathing with pushing down on the medication canister, so you get full benefit from the medication. The only droplets which can benefit you are those you breathe into your bronchial tubes. So hold your breath after inhaling the medication to allow it to spread.

The mist comes out of the puffer in droplets of different sizes. Bigger droplets fall onto your tongue or the back of your throat, and don't get to your lungs, so they don't help. They can give you a bad taste in your mouth, cause hoarseness, and make it more likely that you will develop *thrush,* a common fungal infection. The big drops in the spray may also bump into the smaller drops and combine with them, leaving fewer drops of the right size to get into your lungs.

Because of the need to exactly coordinate your breathing with activating the MDI, and also because of the problems with big droplets, a *spacer* was developed to get small droplets into your bronchial tubes more effectively. A spacer cuts down on side effects from inhaled medication, and is especially important with some inhaled medications. It gets rid of big droplets, and prevents some of the bad taste and sore mouth which may occur with puffer use. We recommend that a spacer be used with all inhalers.

Use of spacers with your puffers may seem like just another hassle to your already-compromised lifestyle. Not necessarily so. Spacers such as the Inspirease™ come in handy carrying pouches that can be disassembled when not in use. It is an easy adjustment that becomes second nature to always use a spacer with MDIs, well worth the effort because spacers deliver medication better than an inhaler alone, right to the lungs.

Sometimes doctors are too busy to take time to show you how to use spacers and

inhalers. If you don't understand, or feel that you aren't doing it right, ask a nurse or respiratory therapist to help you. Or bring it up for discussion and demonstration at a lung support group meeting. *JVT*

Almost all puffers now on the market use Freon, a fluorocarbon which is destroying the ozone layer of the earth. After about 1999, fluorocarbons will be less available, and puffers will have to use a different gas, or medication will have to be delivered in a different way. A new gas called HFA replaces Freon in some inhalers, and new powder inhalers are becoming available in the United States. They are simpler to use and work much more efficiently than the gas inhalers. As fluorocarbons are phased out in the next few years, and as new drugs come to market, inhaled medications will probably change drastically. Talk with your doctor about new options.

Using a metered-dose inhaler

A metered-dose inhaler delivers a dose of medication directly to the lungs, requiring a smaller dose than other delivery methods. The small dose takes effect rapidly, usually within five to ten minutes. Side effects are usually greatly reduced. Inhalers can be used anywhere and at any time, are fairly simple to use and can be used by the elderly and by children as young as five years.

1 Prepare the inhaler.
   If the inhaler is cold, warm it for a few minutes in the palm of your hand.
   If you carry the inhaler in a bag or pocket, inspect it for foreign objects such as a coin or dirt before you use it.

2 Shake the canister well.

3 Remove the cap and position the canister upright, mouthpiece at the bottom.

4 Tilt your head slightly back.

5 Depending on the inhaler type and instructions for use,
   open your mouth with the inhaler one inch away.
   OR Insert the inhaler into your mouth and close your lips around it.
   OR Place the mouthpiece of the spacer in your mouth.

6 Breathe out normally.

7 As you begin a long slow inhalation, press the canister to deliver a puff of medication.

8 Continue to inhale slowly and deeply so that all medication is taken into your lungs.

9 Hold your breath for five to ten seconds at least.

10 If you are using a corticosteroid, rinse your mouth with water or mouthwash.

When you have completed the first delivery, administer repeat puffs as prescribed.

With medications which have an immediate effect, such as beta agonists, wait at least one minute between puffs. This allows the first breath to dilate the airways so that the second puff will be more effective. With preventative medications which have no immediate effect, there is no need to wait between puffs.

Figure 17   Using a metered-dose inhaler

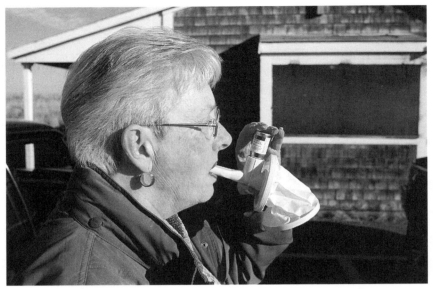

Inhalers can be used anywhere and at any time, are fairly simple to use and can be used by nearly everyone. We recommend that a spacer be used with all inhalers. Jo-Von uses an Inspirease™ spacer with her metered-dose inhaler before going for a walk on the beach.

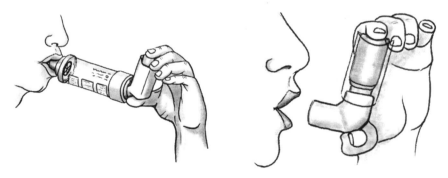

B: Aerochamber™ spacer   C: Without a spacer

Cleaning inhalers and spacers

One advantage of inhalers, in contrast to nebulizers, is that they do not usually need cleaning. If the plastic parts of the inhaler or spacer appear to be soiled, or if the canister is not empty but a mist will not come out, rinse with warm running tap water. Let the components dry thoroughly before using again. You may wash the spacer and mouthpiece in warm dish washing soap, but be sure to rinse thoroughly and let dry.

Change the chamber or diaphragm that comes with some spacers every couple of weeks.

Checking for medicine in the canister

An easy way to check how much medication is left in some canisters is to place the canister in a pan of water.

- If the canister lies horizontally at the bottom of the pan of water, it is close to full.

- If the canister floats with the top near the bottom, it is about 3/4 full.
- If the whole canister floats horizontally at the surface of the water, it is empty.

Not all canisters can be checked in this manner. So check with your doctor or pharmacist to see if you can use this method for your specific inhaler.

Some inhalers contain an exact number of doses, which must be counted.

Powder Inhalers

A different way to provide inhaled medication is in a powder. Powder inhalers do not require gas, such as Freon, nor spacers as you don't have to coordinate your breathing with activating the inhaler. As with the MDIs, some of the medicine goes into your lungs, and some stays in your mouth.

- If the powder is preloaded in an inhaler (Turbohaler™), place the mouthpiece in your mouth and suck in the medication. A single use gives a set amount of medication. Dose is increased by more inhalations.
- If the medication is in a capsule (Rotahaler™), break it open inside the tube provided with the medication. Suck the powder through the end of the tube.

Gas-Driven Nebulizers

Almost all MDI medications are also available in a form for the nebulizer. For people who are very short of breath, or who are unable to coordinate well with an MDI, inhaled medications may be given with a nebulizer. You sit and breathe in the mist continuously through a mouthpiece or mask.

The nebulizer takes at least 10-15 minutes to mix the medicine and use, and extra time to clean.

A gas, usually compressed air, but sometimes oxygen, breaks up liquid medicine into a mist to inhale. The medication is usually mixed with water or salt solution to make it weaker so it can be breathed in over several minutes, in order to get the most effective response.

Nebulizers are available to buy or lease from medical supply houses.

Figure 18   Hand-held nebulizer

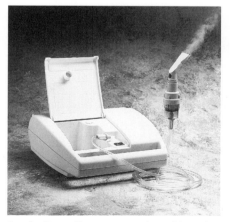

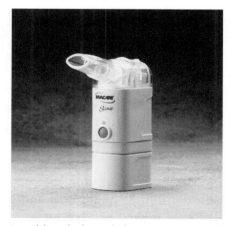

A nebulizer allows you to sit and breathe in the mist continuously through a mouthpiece or mask.

Portable nebulizers help support your active life style.

Using nebulizers

To use a nebulizer with a mouthpiece or mask:

1 Sit up comfortably.

2 Position the mouth piece in your mouth just inside your teeth or apply the mask to your face.

3 During the treatment breathe in through your mouth and out through your mouth or nose, at a normal speed and depth. This allows time for the solution to deposit in your lungs.

4 After every few breaths, exhale completely then take in a deep breath and hold it for five to ten seconds.

5 When you have finished your treatment, if you are having difficulty clearing phlegm, use a controlled coughing technique. See *Coughing* on page 79.

6 If necessary, follow with breathing exercises and postural drainage. See *Postural drainage* on page 78.

7 Clean the equipment as instructed.

Cleaning nebulizers

Keep cleaning solutions in a clean container with a lid. They can be stored for up to one month in the refrigerator.

Never put solution back in the bulk container.

Basic cleaning and sterilization:

- After each use, or as recommended by your doctor, wash the respiratory equipment in warm, *not hot*, clean, soapy water and rinse well. Allow to air dry.
- Once or twice a week after washing and rinsing, soak in bleach and water solution for at least 15 minutes. Then rinse with clean warm water.
- Next, soak in a vinegar and water solution for five minutes or longer. *Do not rinse this solution off.*
- Or, if using quaternary ammonium (Control III™), soak for 10 minutes. *Rinse thoroughly in HOT tap water. DO NOT use soap.*
- After drying, the equipment is ready for use.
- If the nebulizer stops putting out medication, you may need to use a fine wire to clean the tiny nozzle through which the air goes into the medication chamber. If this is not possible, get a new plastic nebulizer.

Bleach and water solutions

For 1 gallon water, use 2 ounces or 1/4 cup bleach.

For 2 quarts water, use 1 ounce or 2 tablespoons bleach.

For 1 quart water, use ½ ounce or 1 tablespoon bleach.

For 1 pint water, use 2 teaspoons bleach.

Vinegar and water solutions

1 pint 5% white vinegar to 1 pint water.

½ cup 5% white vinegar to ½ pint water.

Quaternary ammonium

Quaternary ammonium compounds such as Control III™ cost less than vinegar, have no odor, and can be purchased through a home care company or a drugstore.

Do not exceed the recommended number of uses and lengths of time for use, to avoid degrading the nebulizer plastics.

In a food-grade plastic container, mix:

1 tablespoon (1/2 oz.) Control III to 1 quart water.

Keep covered when not in use. Do not reuse longer than 14 days.

Test solution daily with test strips. If solution is visibly dirty, or falls below 1,000 ppm (parts per million), dump it and make a fresh solution.

Normal saline solution

Can be purchased as Bronchosol™ or other brands.

For 1 cup or 8 ounces of distilled water, use ¼ teaspoon *non-iodized* salt.

For 2 cups or 16 ounces of distilled water use ½ teaspoon *non-iodized* salt.

Buy distilled water at your grocery or pharmacy.

- Boil the water and salt gently for five minutes in a clean ceramic pan or heat in the microwave.
- When cooled, place in a clean tightly-covered container and store in the refrigerator. Do not keep longer than one week.

Medications for COPD

Some of the COPD medications currently available in the United States are listed in the following pages. If you don't find your particular medications in these lists, ask your doctor what categories they belong to, so you can see what effects they should have.

You may be on a number of inhaled medications, each with a different action. A different medication is often added rather than going to a higher dose, to reduce side effects and relieve your symptoms more completely.

Bronchodilators

Bronchodilators open up or dilate the bronchial tubes for easy passage of air. They relax the muscle around the bronchial tubes so that it will not be in spasm. When the muscle spasm relaxes, the inside of the bronchial tube is wider making it easier to breathe and cough up mucus. Bronchodilators are inhaled from a puffer device or a nebulizer. They are usually liquid, but some powder and pill preparations are available.

Quick-acting beta-agonist bronchodilators

Beta agonists such as those listed are the most common bronchodilators in use today. They get their group name from the way they work, stimulating an area of the cell called the *beta receptor*. These agents usually start working within a couple of minutes. As they usually don't last very long, they can be used every few hours if needed. In general, they are used because COPD symptoms are getting worse, for increased shortness of breath, wheezing or cough. If exacerbation is

Table 3: Beta-agonist bronchodilators: quick acting

Generic Name	Trade Name
metaproterenol	Alupent™, Metaprel™
albuterol	Proventil™ Ventolin™ Rotahaler™ (albuterol powder)
terbutaline	Brethaire™
pirbuterol	Maxair™
bitolterol	Tornalate™
isoetharine	Bronkometer™
epinephrine	Primatene™ (not a good drug for COPD and not recommended)

going on, or if the disease is severe, these medications may be used regularly, as often as every three to four hours. They are also used before vigorous exercise to prevent shortness of breath during or after the exercise.

Several different firms make beta agonists, to be used in metered dose inhalers, as powder inhalations or for nebulizers.

Studies have not shown many differences between the more commonly prescribed medications released in the last 15 years. Medications available before that, such as epinephrine (Primatene) or adrenaline and isoproterenol lasted a much shorter length of time and were much more likely to cause side effects. Now they are rarely used.

Side effects of commonly-used, inhaled beta-2 agonists include anxiety and occasional rapid heart rate or dizziness. For most, these side effects are mild and tend to disappear shortly after use of the medication.

Long-acting bronchodilators

Table 4: Beta-agonist and anti-cholinergic bronchodilators: medium to long acting

Generic Name	Trade Name
ipratropium bromide (medium)	Atrovent™
ipratropium and albuterol (quick onset, medium length)	Combivent™
salmeterol (long)	Serevent™
formoterol (long)	Not yet available in the U.S.

Salmeterol and formoterol are very long-acting, lasting about 12 hours. Salmeterol is available in the U.S., packaged as Serevent, a spray inhaler. Formoterol will be available soon as a powder inhaler. Both medications may cause either shakiness or tremor, or increase anxiety. With regular use, they are very effective for long-lasting relief of shortness of breath. They need to be used regularly, every 12 hours, but as they do not work right away, you need to keep quick-acting medicines at hand.

Serevent (salmeterol) is available only as an inhaler, although nebulizer medication is planned.

Another important bronchodilator, recommended for regular use in COPD, is inhaled ipratropium bromide (Atrovent). It may slow progression of the COPD, so it is recommended by many pulmonary physicians. This medication does not work quite as quickly as the beta-2 agonists, taking about 30 minutes, but its effects last longer. It may be used as needed, but more often is recommended on a schedule.

Ipratropium is available as an inhaler or as a liquid for nebulizer. The most common side effect of ipratropium is spasmodic cough, which is usually relieved by stopping the medication. If a high dose of ipratropium or atropine is used it may cause difficulty in urinating, particularly in men. Ipratropium may be mixed with albuterol or one of the other quick-acting bronchodilators in a nebulizer.

A new inhaler, Combivent, combining ipratropium with albuterol is also available for more convenient dosing.

Corticosteroids or Steroids

Corticosteroids are different from anabolic steroids used by athletes to promote muscle growth and strength. Medical use of steroids, when taken as prescribed, does not damage the liver and does not produce heart disease which is seen as a result of high anabolic-steroid use in athletes.

Corticosteroids are frequently used in the treatment of COPD. They are powerful medications, effective in the treatment of acute episodes of worsening shortness of breath, sometimes when nothing else seems to work. They have been given a bad name partly due to fear of their side effects, and partly due to confusion between corticosteroids and anabolic steroids.

Corticosteroids must be used on a regular basis. They are strictly preventative, and have no immediate benefit.

Inhaled corticosteroids

Inhaled corticosteroids are fairly new medications, and safest when compared to oral or injected steroids, because they have fewer side effects outside the mouth, airways and lungs. However, they may cause osteoporosis, or bone loss.

All corticosteroids have the potential for quite significant side-effects, depending on dosage more than any other factor. Inhaled steroid dosages are much smaller than oral or injected dosages. However, long-term use of even inhaled steroids has the potential to cause problems. Inhaled corticosteroids have direct effects on the upper airway, including the mouth, tongue and vocal cords, where they may cause soreness, hoarseness, or overgrowth of the common fungus, thrush. These side effects are less likely if you use a spacer device, and when you rinse your mouth after each set of inhalations. You don't need to wait between puffs.

The inhaled steroid cuts down on chronic inflammation, preventing further lung damage so the COPD may stabilize. In fact, some studies have shown that using inhaled steroids prevents progression of COPD, at least over the short term.

Over several years, inhaled steroids may affect your eyes, so if you are taking inhaled steroids get regular eye exams to detect early cataracts or glaucoma.

Some of the newer, stronger inhaled steroids may cause the body to stop normal production of steroids, so that when you stop taking them, or if you have a severe illness, it is possible to suffer from steroid shortage. This possibility is being studied, and your doctor needs to be aware of steroids you are taking in any form.

Table 5: Preventative medications: steroid liquid and powder inhalers

Generic Name	Trade Name
triamcinolone 100 micrograms	Azmacort™
beclomethasone 42 micrograms	Vanceril™ Beclovent™
beclomethasone 84 micrograms	Vanceril DS™
flunisolone 250 micrograms/puff	Aerobid M™
fluticazone 220, 110, or 44 micrograms	Flovent™
budesonide 200mcg (powder)	Pulmicort Turbohaler™

Dose comparisons

Overall, inhaled steroids are safe because they are administered in small doses. For example:

- A small pill of a common steroid, *prednisone* (Deltasone™ and other names), delivers 5,000 micrograms or 5 milligrams.
- One puff of a common inhaled corticosteroid, *beclomethasone* (Vanceril DS), gives 84 micrograms per puff, but less into the lung where it is absorbed. Using a fairly standard regimen of beclomethasone of four puffs daily gives a total dose of 336 micrograms. It would take over 60 puffs daily to equal one prednisone tablet.

There are two reasons that a small dose can be used in the inhaled form of steroid.

- The drug goes only to the mouth and the lung, so it is not wasted.
- The inhaled steroid is used for prevention, not treatment.

Inhaled steroids do not correct a severe exacerbation of wheezing COPD, and as for almost all preventatives, inhaled steroids must be taken regularly while you are stable. Although the newer more potent inhaled steroids are sometimes used to treat an acute attack, they should only be used during an attack following your doctor's instructions.

Systemic Corticosteroids as Pills or Injections

Corticosteroid pills or injections treat increased shortness of breath, increased cough or other acute exacerbations and symptoms of lung disease. In general, due to side-effects, doctors try to have you on steroids for the shortest possible time: a large dose initially, rapidly cut down as you improve over several days. Treatment is usually complete within one to two weeks.

Steroids have strong anti-inflammatory properties and will stop bronchospasm (wheezing), reduce swelling of the air tubes and cut down on the production of mucus. Whether an injected steroid or pills are used depends on how ill you are, whether intestinal difficulties are present, how high a dose you need, and how long the medication is to continue. Most doctors avoid chronic or long-term use of steroids, because of their side effects.

When you start on corticosteroids during an acute episode, you may be unable to stop them because of continuing shortness of breath. Getting you off steroids needs your cooperation and understanding, particularly if shortness-of-breath increases as the steroid dosage is decreased or tapered. Intermittent slow-release steroids given by injection are as harmful as an equivalent dose taken daily by mouth.

Side Effects of Corticosteroids

Many positive and negative side effects are associated with use of oral or injected steroids:

- Improved sense of well-being
- Improved appetite
- Fluid retention
- Weight gain
- Rounding of the face
- Changes in mood
- Increased blood pressure.

These side effects will go away when you stop taking the steroid. However, *never stop the steroid on your own.* Always consult your doctor.

Long-term side effects may not clear when the medication is stopped. These include:

- Development of diabetes
- Weight gain
- Osteoporosis (thinning of the bones)
- Cataracts
- Myopathy (muscle weakness).

WARNING: **People who have been on steroids long enough to develop these side effects generally need a very gradual decrease in dose to prevent *Addison's disease*, due to a lack of corticosteroids.**

If you have questions about the use of corticosteroids, ask your doctor.

Non-steroid Anti-inflammatory Inhalers: Preventative

Table 6: Non-steroid inhalers: preventative (for asthma and allergy)

Generic Name	Trade Name
cromolyn	Intal™
nedocromil	Tilade™

Cromolyn is a very safe medication, only rarely causing spasmodic cough, but is rarely prescribed for COPD. In people who wheeze frequently and have a diagnosis of asthma or allergies in addition to the COPD, it may be tried on a regular basis for a few weeks to see if it helps. In people who develop wheezing with exercise, it may be used 15 to 30 minutes before exercising. A newer medication, Nedocromil (Tilade), is not frequently used in COPD, but seems to relieve spasms of cough in some people. These medicines should not be used for acute or rapid onset episodes.

Anti-inflammatory Pills

Table 7: Anti-inflammatory pills: preventative (for asthma and allergy)

Generic Name	Trade Name
zafirlukast	Accolate™
montelukast	Singulair™

Two new asthma medicines, montelukast, taken once daily, and zafirlukast, taken twice daily, may also be useful in COPD. They prevent inflammation which may cause damage to the bronchial tubes. It is hoped that these pills will help prevent acute attacks of bronchitis and wheezing if used regularly.

Nasal Inhalers

Table 8: Steroids: nasal inhalers

Generic Name	Trade Name
fluticazone	Flonase™
triamcinolone	Nasalcort™
beclomethasone	Beconase AQ, Beconase™ Vancenase AQ, Vancenase™
flunisolide	Nasalide, Nasarel™

Table 9: Non-steroids: nasal inhalers

Generic Name	Trade Name
cromolyn	Nasalcrom™
ipratropium	Atrovent™

Nasal inhalers are used to treat and prevent chronic nasal stuffiness and drainage and thus prevent *chronic sinusitis*. A common problem that occurs with COPD is *chronic rhinitis* or *sinusitis*, inflammation of the nose, causing nasal or post-nasal drip, nasal stuffiness, hoarseness, and blocked nasal passages. If rhinitis is severe, it may cause the sinuses to become inflamed or infected. The reasons for these problems are related to allergies and also to direct irritation. Unfortunately, the nasal problems can last a long time after the direct irritation has cleared up, becoming *perennial rhinitis*.

Treatment is important, as nasal drip and blocking may worsen lung problems. The tables list nasal sprays which may be used regularly to subdue symptoms. There are many different nasal sprays available without a prescription; some can harm the nose if used regularly, so consult your doctor before using one.

Use nasal inhalers once or twice a day. Many are the same as those that treat lung symptoms.

Theophylline

Theophylline has been used in treatment of lung disease for many years. Its major purpose in COPD is to reduce bronchospasm, which relieves shortness of breath. It may also help the diaphragm to work more effectively, preventing fatigue with increased activity. Unfortunately, it acts in so many different ways that it has about as many ill effects as good. Because of its side effects, it is used less frequently than inhaled medications.

Theophylline is most frequently administered as sustained-release pills or capsules. In acute illness, it may be given intravenously. As theophylline takes time to build up in the blood stream to a therapeutic level, adjustment may be necessary, with blood testing to monitor your blood level. The blood level is almost always measured when you are admitted to a hospital or after a dosage adjustment, particularly an increase in dosage. If the blood level goes too high it will need to be reduced quickly to avoid side effects. This is why it is important for you to stay in contact with your doctor.

Some people cannot tolerate theophylline. A major side effect is anxiety, which may lead to tremulousness and insomnia, even in therapeutic doses and with normal blood levels. Other frequent side effects include nausea sometimes with vomiting, stomach cramps, and diarrhea. These symptoms usually improve with dose reduction. Mild side effects will usually go away within a few hours or a day after a dosage reduction. At times, a single dose daily given at the time of maximal difficulty breathing can be tolerated and will be helpful.

Some side effects occur with a very high level of medication: irregular heart beat, severe headaches and even seizures. Call your doctor if these symptoms develop. You may simply require an adjustment in dose.

Expectorants and Mucolytics

Table 10: Expectorant and mucolytic agents

Generic Name	Trade Name
guaifenesin	Humibid™, Tussi-organidin™

Expectorants and mucolytics help liquefy secretions and allow you to cough up mucus more easily. One of the best expectorants is water. Drinking an adequate amount of water, one quart per day, will make clearing phlegm easier, which may lead to improved breathing. However, water intake may be limited by your doctor because of other problems such as heart disease.

A common medication in this category is guaifenesin.

Antibiotics

Antibiotics are used to treat infections caused by bacteria. Doctors suspect bacterial infection when a person is coughing up increased amounts of sputum, often discolored yellow or green, and particularly with a low-grade temperature. Antibiotics are not helpful in treating viral infections, which may also produce sputum discoloration.

There are many types of antibiotics for different infection-causing bacteria. Sometimes a specimen of phlegm is collected to see what type of bacteria are present, so that the correct antibiotic can be prescribed. Infection may clear without antibiotic treatment. Tremendous variation in the price of antibiotics may make a difference in the antibiotic prescribed.

Some people have an allergic reaction to a particular drug, so if you know that you have an allergy, let your doctor know. For emergency purposes it would be wise to get Medic Alert identification to let medical personnel know about your condition. See *Organizations* on page 237.

You may have read or heard that bacteria all over the world are becoming resistant to more and more antibiotics. This means that some antibiotics will not kill the target bacteria, even when they are given in appropriate dosages for the correct amount of time. This has made many doctors reluctant to treat people with antibiotics just because the sputum is discolored, without other evidence of infection. Antibiotic prescription in the future will be more cautious, for fear of increasing antibiotic resistance.

Antifungals

Antifungal medications are used occasionally in people with COPD, especially if high doses of inhaled or oral steroids are prescribed. Thrush is treated with a gargle or pills containing an antifungal agent. Less commonly, a fungal infection may reach the lungs, particularly with high doses of steroids for a long time.

Severe fungal infection in the lungs is diagnosed by bronchoscopy or surgery and requires extended treatment. People who have weak immune systems, for example after a lung transplant, may need continuous antifungal treatment.

Antivirals

Antiviral treatment is available to treat influenza (the flu), although prevention by yearly vaccination is the best course. Antiviral medicines can shorten illness and reduce severity, but to be effective, medication must start as soon as possible after the first symptoms. At times, medication is started after an exposure to the flu but before symptoms are evident.

New medications to treat a cold are coming to market, such as nasal sprays to shorten the time a cold lasts and decrease the symptoms.

Diuretics

Diuretics are commonly referred to as *water pills*, because they help to eliminate excess water from the body, reducing swelling and lowering high blood pressure. In people with severe COPD, low oxygen level may lead to weakening of the heart, swelling of the ankles, and swelling of other parts of the body, including the abdomen. This may result in increasing shortness of breath. Treatment includes correcting the low oxygen level and giving diuretics to reduce swelling.

Diuretics should be taken in the morning, to avoid waking up at night to urinate. They may be taken as pills once a day, or given intravenously. Diuretics are more effective if taken with meals, when the largest load of salt and water is presented to the body.

Some diuretics may also eliminate large amounts of potassium, so it is common for a potassium supplement to be ordered or for your doctor to suggest that you increase your intake of certain foods high in potassium. Bananas, lima beans, split peas, sweet potatoes, fresh spinach, dates, raisins, dried fruits, orange juice, salmon, bacon, and beef are all excellent sources. Signs of low potassium include muscle weakness and cramps. If you have these signs see your doctor for a simple blood test to confirm low potassium. A diuretic which does not produce as much loss of potassium, such as *hydrochlorothiazide/triamterene* is often prescribed.

Diuretics can also produce loss of sodium and other essential chemicals. While you are taking diuretics, ask your doctor to periodically check the level of these substances in your blood.

Vaccines for Influenza and Pneumonia

Almost all elderly people and people with chronic diseases such as COPD are highly encouraged to get yearly influenza vaccine or *flu shots*.

Most years these shots are effective, but effectiveness depends on the vaccine development process. Most viruses which produce epidemics in North America and Europe have previously done so in Asia (Beijing Flu, Taiwan Flu). The Centers for Disease Control in Atlanta develops vaccine for the United States to protect from whatever viruses were in Asia six months earlier. But sometimes new viruses occur in the U.S. without first showing up in Asia, and sometimes the viruses change. Therefore, there is no guarantee, even with vaccination, that you will avoid the flu. If you do get it, however, chances are good that you will have a milder case if you've had the shot.

The flu shot cannot cause flu. Side effects of the shots may include redness or pain at the injection site, but developing a cold or flu-like symptoms after vaccination is usually due to exposure to an infected person while getting the flu shot, or at about the same time.

The pneumonia vaccine, *Pneumovax*, was developed to prevent pneumonias caused by the pneumococcus bacteria, which can cause severe, even fatal pneumonia. After receiving Pneumovax, your body is able to make antibodies against the pneumococcus bacteria. These antibodies, in people with COPD, appear to remain at high levels for five to ten years or longer, so injections at about ten-year intervals are usually recommended. This vaccine can cause increased soreness and swelling at the injection site if given too soon after the last injection, because of the high antibody levels still present in your body.

If you have COPD, get other routine vaccinations, such as tetanus, just as anyone else of your age would do.

Other Treatments

Clearing Mucus

A major problem with COPD is increased amount and thickness of mucus. Mucus becomes difficult to cough up, may plug air passages, and must be cleared periodically. If an expectorant such as guaifenesin is not successful, your phsyician may decide to try chest physiotherapy.

Chest physiotherapy

Use these techniques only when needed for increased thick mucus that resists coming up with coughing, but not after a meal, when the stomach is full. Not all lung areas may need drainage.

Chest physiotherapy is most effective and least likely to cause increased spasms of cough if you use a bronchodilator 30 minutes before, to open the airways and allow better drainage. You learn quickly which areas need chest physiotherapy, the usual amount of fluid brought up, and your feelings following treatment.

Chest physiotherapy includes *postural drainage, chest percussion* or *vibration*, and *cough*. Your doctor and trial and error can help you decide what's best.

Postural drainage

Postural drainage is lying in different positions in order to drain different lobes of your lungs. At times, it is difficult to tolerate the angles needed for drainage, particularly head-down positions. A tilt board or pillows on a bed, couch or floor can create more comfortable drainage positions. Each position should be maintained for five to ten minutes, or longer, to clear secretions. Postural drainage may be carried out as often as four times a day, although it is rarely necessary that often.

Figure 19   Postural drainage

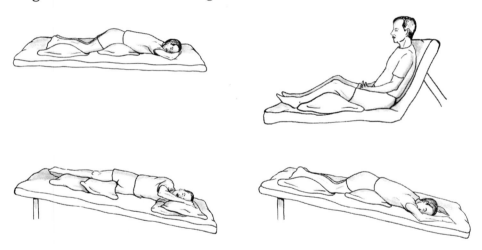

Some of the positions your doctor can prescribe in order to drain different lobes of your lungs.

Percussion

Percussion and vibration may be used to dislodge mucus during postural drainage. Get someone with training to do percussion; the instructions for percussion and vibration are addressed to the person giving these treatments.

Percussion is applied by striking the chest area with cupped hands or by using a mechanical percussor. If you are giving this treatment, deliver percussion about five times per second, for one to five minutes over the lung zone that needs draining. Place a towel over the chest area to protect sensitive skin. There are no definitive guidelines for how hard to strike the chest.

> **WARNING:** **The person doing percussion should be trained in this treatment. Be cautious, particularly with people who may have very brittle bones which may break.**

Vibration

Vibration is another technique that can be used to assist in mucus drainage. Apply downward shaking pressure about 10 to 15 times a second, over the lung zone to be drained. Mechanical vibrations can be used.

Coughing

Coughing can expel excess mucus from the larger airways. Following a deep breath, try to cough while you use your throat muscles to keep the mucus from coming out. This helps mucus move to the larger air tubes, where it may be easier to clear out.

Avoiding Irritants

The same things which bother people with asthma also bother people with COPD. People with COPD are bothered by dust and fumes. Avoid such irritating substances, especially if you wheeze. Cigarette and pipe smoke, paint fumes, cleaning solutions, perfumes and other cosmetics, dust, pets, cold air, may cause worsening of COPD.

Avoiding irritants takes some planning. Avoiding irritants at home should be easiest. *It is critical that nobody smokes in your home.* If someone smokes, beg them to do it only outside. Going into another room does not help, as smoke circulates through the house. Do not hesitate to put a NO SMOKING! sign on the door of your home.

- Vacuum the house at least weekly. If you do not have a vacuum with a very good filtration/dustcatching system, buy one.
- Avoid carpets and upholstered furniture, especially in the bedroom, in order to prevent dust from accumulating. Cats are very likely to cause allergy.
- Clear mold out of the house, especially from the bathroom, kitchen and basement, and stop water leaks to prevent mold from returning.
- Have someone else do major house cleaning or emptying out old dusty closets, at a time when you are out of the house for several hours.
- At work or in public, avoid places such as malls where smoking is allowed.
- Avoid manufacturing and petrochemical processing centers, as they release fumes.
- Stay away from public gatherings where people smoke.
- Stay away from stores that are heavily perfumed.
- Stay indoors if there are air pollution warnings.

Supplements to Treatment

One of the most common complaints of people with COPD is that their doctor dismisses their complaints or symptoms, simply because they are elderly. A common response is "For your age, you are doing as well as can be expected." The doctor seems to have no idea that hope is removed by dismissing concerns. Even if there is little hope, it is best to leave room for the possibility of improvement. People don't want to be lied to, but neither do they wish to be fluffed off because of age. People do improve in miraculous, unexpected ways, in spite of what the doctor may think. Hope should never be taken away.

However doctors cannot feel what you feel, and do not know your concerns first-hand. They can only know what they have learned from text books and lectures, and from what they have observed. They haven't "walked in your shoes."

Encouragement, emotional and spiritual support play vital roles in the wellness of lung patients. As there is only so much support that your doctor can provide, look to your family, friends, and most importantly, to yourself.

The optimum condition is stability for anyone with COPD. If you are no longer getting worse, but managing to hold your own, you are probably stable. Your doctor will be able to tell you.

Some of the most valuable things I have learned about managing COPD and its symptoms have been from some of my fellow COPD sufferers in the support group, or by developing solutions on my own. I've also gathered a lot of information from research.

A lot of my time and energy is devoted to holding onto my fragile stable status, and I constantly look for ways to enhance and support my doctor's prescribed treatment.

Nothing that I do is contrary to what Dr. Mohr prescribes. Each undertaking helps my course of treatment work even better, and receives Dr. Mohr's "blessing". We are often surprised by my accomplishments. With a stable condition, I am able to work every day, and travel for business and pleasure, although I haven't yet ventured on a foreign jaunt. My life is full, and busy, and rich. And I intend to keep it so, just as long as I can manage it. The alternative is simply unacceptable.

Alternatives and Supplements to Medicine

You should each follow whatever philosophies and methodologies are available to help in your battle against lung disease. What works best for one may not work at all for another. Check with your doctor to be sure that a new course that you are following on your own is not in conflict with your prescribed treatment.

Mindful Meditation

As developed in the Buddhist traditions of Asia, *mindful meditation* is moment-to-moment awareness, allowing for development of new control and wisdom, based on capacities for relaxation, paying attention, awareness, and insight. You focus on your breath and allow yourself to return to your breathing when you become aware of thoughts. This can be self-taught, or taken in a class. It is an alternative to medicine for reducing stress, and if practiced successfully, can help alleviate symptoms.

Dr. Kabat-Zinn's book, *Full Catastrophe Living*, discusses the personal commitment required to practice mindful meditation each day. "The basic idea is to create an island of being in the sea of constant doing in which our lives are usually immersed, a time in which we allow all the doing to stop." Mindfulness allows life's problems to be seen more clearly and objectively through the lens of a clear mind. It is a way of introducing simplicity to your life, and of allowing healing and well-being as natural progressions of meditation.

Meditation is not a passive process; it requires effort to fully focus, and to remain genuinely calm and nonreactive. By concentrating on your own breathing, you can begin to regulate your body systems and let go of thoughts and reminders of pain that race through your brain. It is an effective way of leaving that busyness, and moving on to relaxation and peacefulness.

My experience with mindful meditation began many years before I became ill. I studied meditation, then Yoga, and later mindful meditation on my own, as a young adult. I learned to get in touch with my own body, to scan it, and to develop relaxation techniques that helped me greatly in my stressful professional life. I undertook the study of meditation specifically to reduce stress and pain, although at the time, most of my pain was emotional.

Now I have returned to mindful meditation to help me through chronic illness. I have been able to significantly lower my high blood pressure, nearly eliminating medication for the condition. My blood pressure readings now are within a safe range, controlled through daily mindful meditation, and a small dose of medicine. This has been followed closely by the endocrinologist who treats me for diabetes and hypertension.

Meditation has helped me through many phases of anxiety and trauma of my battles with COPD and diabetes. The times that I set aside each day for meditation are special gifts to myself, of serenity and peace, free from pain and worry. By concentrating on my breathing for a few minutes, I am able to slip into an altered state of consciousness, opening up my body, mind and soul to awareness and the warm healing powers of a life without stress, at least for a while.

Visualizing

Visualizing during meditation helps to focus. It helps to discard bothersome thoughts and preoccupations and allows you to concentrate on something pleasant. It is a place where you can sit quietly and focus on healing your body. *The Magic Shop*, by Helen Graham, is an excellent book for learning visualization techniques. These techniques are often taught as part of meditation training. Librarians and good bookstores can recommend other helpful books.

I concentrate on bringing the place and the moment alive inside my brain. After each visualization, I feel rested, comforted, happy and well, or at least free from pain.

I visualize a snow-covered mountain in the Himalayas, and can bring to myself the strength and support that is a mountain, and the clean air that surrounds it. I become the mountain, firmly joined to the ground while reaching to the heavens. My breathing is deep, regular, and effortless. I often visualize a garden that I particularly loved in Ireland, with soft light, winding walkways, a stone bench by a quiet, reflective pool ringed with blossoms, colors, scents and textures. Sometimes I visualize a beach that I loved in Tahiti where I hear the crash of surf as I bask in the warmth of the sunshine, and the sweet smells of plumeria and the salt of the ocean.

Yoga

Yoga is relaxing and generates blood circulation. It also promotes concentration and focused breathing. It can help to quickly assimilate the techniques of meditation. Yoga is a form of exercise that promotes wellness and fitness through stretching and muscle toning, including the muscles used for breathing. It helps if your body is limber enough to be able to go through the various movements and positions of yoga. But, even with some impairment, Yoga can be done by almost everyone.

Yoga can be self-taught but it is better to sign up for some instruction, either private or in a small class, in order to learn it correctly. If you are doing an exercise or movement wrong it can cause more harm than good.

One tip for Yoga and T'ai Chi: if it hurts, stop. Yoga should not be painful. You are pushing too far, or doing something wrong, if an exercise becomes painful. Learn to listen to your body's distress signals, even in the practice of Yoga and other forms of meditation.

T'ai Chi Chuan

Anyone, even people with lung disease, can do T'ai Chi. It is not strenuous. You focus on your breathing and your moves as you slowly and smoothly turn and change positions to stretch both mind and body. T'ai Chi teaches self-control, concentration and focus, and coordination; and it improves balance. T'ai Chi is another ancient Chinese form of exercise refined to an art. It is a series of slow and smooth choreographed movements, which help to stretch and tone muscles. There is a rhythm and flow to T'ai Chi Chuan that makes it both beautiful to watch, and fulfilling to do. There is something cleansing about it.

The basic movements of T'ai Chi are simple to learn, and just require practice. More complicated series of exercises require daily practice, are challenging, and tend to keep you more interested over a long period of time.

You can usually locate a T'ai Chi instructor through your local gymnasium, or through a Council on Aging.

We put together a special class of beginning students through our support group, which was great because we all had the same basic restrictions, all with lung disease. Later, people from the Orleans Senior Center joined our group, and you could not tell the difference between those with COPD and healthy folks from the Senior Center. It is easily learned, and very enjoyable. When you have lung disease it is important to spend your limited energy on activities that feed the soul, as well as doing satisfying physical exercise. T'ai Chi does both.

The Way to Stay Stable

Following are simple but important rules to keep stable in your battle with COPD. These are *supplements* to your treatment, not replacements, although some alternatives are suggested. These points may seem simple and fundamental. They are. But they are easy to forget, as you get caught up in your often-frustrating efforts each day. So this list is a reminder, even to the experienced and knowledgeable patient, of some of the things to do to avoid complications and infections.

- Avoid breathing irritating things such as dust, fumes, and polluted air.
- Stay indoors when air pollution and pollen counts are high.
- Religiously avoid cigarette smoke, first or second hand.

- Follow your doctor's instructions on the use of medications.
- Get an annual flu shot.
- Get a vaccination against pneumonia every eight to ten years.
- Avoid crowds, especially during flu season when respiratory infections are everywhere.
- Eat well and maintain proper nutrition.
- Avoid extreme temperatures.
- Make exercise conditioning, even a modest program, part of your daily life.

The last point, exercise conditioning, may be the most difficult, if exertion of any kind sends you gasping to the nearest chair. But exercise is an essential part of treatment. People who follow a regular, sustained exercise program usually improve their physical abilities. This helps in performing daily and other activities with less shortness of breath. See *Exercise* on page 121, and *Exercise Programs* on page 137.

This is most certainly hardest for me. It is tough finding energy or time to exercise, especially since I work a minimum of 40 hours a week. But I am committed to four or five sessions a week. It would be much better every day, and I know it, but I don't usually do it. Depending on the way I feel, just to get bathed and dressed and to work on time requires great effort. By the time the work day has ended for me, I am so exhausted that exercise is the last thing on my mind.

Don't do as I do, allowing pressures of work or anything else to push aside your commitment to exercise. It is a vicious circle. We need to exercise, but it takes energy to do so. We have no energy. We are chronically fatigued, but we need to strengthen our muscles to breathe more easily. Our bodies need conditioning to provide us with the extra strength.

Encourage your doctor to refer you for pulmonary rehabilitation. This will help you get started exercising. If you don't have a great support group like Jo-Von's, pulmonary rehab will help you meet other people with COPD. You may make new friends.

RC, BN, JVT

5　Supplemental Oxygen

Supplemental oxygen is not habit-forming, but needs to be used according to your doctor's recommendations. For people with chronic bronchitis or emphysema, it may be prescribed for sleep, during exercise, or 24 hours a day. Present medical knowledge supports continuous use of supplemental oxygen for people with a low oxygen value at rest in their usual state of health. Oxygen flow rates may be adjusted for periods of increased activity and sleep.

Health and Lifestyle Benefits

The benefits of oxygen therapy have been shown to include an improved survival rate as well as improvements in intellectual and emotional functioning and exercise tolerance. Working with your doctor, respiratory therapist, and home care provider, you can learn how to use different types of oxygen storage and delivery for improving your ability to move around, improving your level of activity, for extending your freedom, and generally improving the quality of your life.

I have been on supplemental oxygen around the clock for 10 years. I'm still loving life and you can, too. It saddens me to see newly diagnosed patients react with fear and resignation when supplemental oxygen is prescribed. Don't be frightened. I can tell you from experience that supplemental oxygen provides far more benefits than negatives. Extra oxygen helps lessen fatigue, helps with more energy, and may help with shortness of breath. Oxygen will improve and extend your life.

While you may feel self-conscious at first, wearing your cannula and toting a system, it is amazing how quickly you will adjust. When you are comfortable, people around you adjust. You may be surprised how quickly the concern of others about your nasal cannula disappears. Relax, forget about the oxygen, and after a few months using your equipment, it will become second nature and settle into a routine.

Great strides have been made in oxygen equipment, especially in providing maximum time with minimum hassle and discomfort. The wonderful thing about these products is that they open up new worlds for us. We no longer have to stay at home close to the electric concentrator, and turn down invitations.

I recently used the Oxylite system and was pleased to discover that this tiny portable system provides up to ten hours at two liters per minute (lpm), compared to my regular portable which supplies only seven hours. Those extra hours give me access to new places and events. Now I can take a boat trip from Cape Cod to Nantucket for the whole day, enjoy browsing and shopping, poking around in the galleries, having lunch at one of the quaint restaurants by the sea, and still have plenty of oxygen to get me all the way home again.

My point is that your prescription for supplemental oxygen should not restrict you to a heavily-compromised lifestyle. In fact it's quite possible to lead a very active life because of the benefits you get from oxygen. Work with your oxygen provider to determine which of the portable systems will best serve your needs, your wishes to stay physically active and involved with life. Don't be intimidated by the equipment—it is all very easy to use.

For those newly diagnosed, and for those who have been on oxygen for a while, and have become resigned to staying at home, the new equipment can give you amazing freedom of movement and get you out and about once more.

Determining the Need

People with severe disease or acute illness may have lower than normal oxygen level in the blood and need extra oxygen. The purpose of supplemental oxygen is to return the amount of oxygen in the blood to a normal level. Deciding when to administer supplemental oxygen is usually done either by drawing arterial blood gases or by oximetry.

Abnormal values have been arrived at by consensus among medical experts and are used in the United States for reimbursement by Medicare.

The amount of oxygen in the blood is measured as the *oxygen partial pressure.* Normal value depends on the altitude, but at sea level in an older person the blood oxygen value is typically above 80 millimeters of mercury. In a person with COPD, an oxygen pressure below 55 is abnormal enough that extra oxygen is usually prescribed.

The amount of oxygen which is bound to hemoglobin, the red pigment in the blood, is called the *oxygen saturation* or *saturation.* A normal level is above 96%. Saturation values at or below 87% are abnormal and enough extra oxygen is prescribed to get the saturation level above 90%.

If an abnormal oxygen level is found during an acute illness, then after recovery another set of blood gases is drawn to see if oxygen is needed on a long-term basis. In a person who has other disease, particularly heart disease, supplemental oxygen may be administered even with a higher oxygen level.

Testing Oxygen Needs

Arterial blood gas or oximetry testing is most commonly done during a daytime office visit. If you have certain symptoms suggesting periodic oxygen lows, your doctor may request monitoring of your oxygen saturation level at night, while you are asleep. If your resting oxygen level is normal but you are very short of breath during exercise, your oxygen level can be checked while you walk a treadmill or ride an exercise bicycle. If the test demonstrates low oxygen level, supplemental oxygen will be started or increased, and your oxygen level will be rechecked to confirm your oxygen needs, or that adjustments are needed.

Your Prescription

Your oxygen prescription sets the oxygen flow rate you need, possibly with different rates for resting, exercise, and sleep. Flow rates are measured in liters per minute, and usually range from one to six liters per minute (lpm).

Prescriptions for oxygen should be filled by qualified respiratory therapists or other qualified people working for companies that specialize in home care and durable medical equipment. They will provide you with equipment, supplies, and oxygen, and should be able to demonstrate use, answer your questions, and help to solve any problems.

There are several types of oxygen systems. For an active lifestyle outside the home you may need a small, portable system that can provide many hours of oxygen. When you are at home you may need only a stationary system. Or you may use a device which concentrates oxygen from the air to provide a continuous source.

When your oxygen flow rates are established, you need to estimate how long oxygen can be supplied by various systems, depending on their capacity and your needs. To extend the length of time for a cylinder you can use a conserving system. See *Oxygen Conserving Equipment* on page 97, and *Selecting a Conserving Device* on page 99.

Your home care or medical equipment supplier will be able to help you figure out what you need.

Oxygen Storage Systems

There are two main categories of oxygen storage systems:

- stationary or base systems
- portable systems.

They are combined with oxygen breathing equipment to deliver supplemental oxygen as and when it is needed. See *Oxygen Breathing Equipment* on page 96.

Stationary systems provide a large source of oxygen but restrict movement to your home or office. Some systems can be used to fill portable systems. Although cost may limit your options, you should be able to find a system or combination of systems to meet your needs.

Warnings About Oxygen Use

WARNING: **Stay at least eight (8) feet away from an open flame while using oxygen. Do not use oxygen while cooking with an open flame such as gas appliances, or gas or charcoal-fired barbecue.**

WARNING: **Never smoke while using oxygen, nor around someone using oxygen.**

Put a sign on the door of every room where oxygen is in use:
OXYGEN IN USE
NO SMOKING

WARNING: Never use petroleum-based face creams or ointments, such as Vaseline. Use only water-based creams, lotions, and cosmetics.

WARNING: Never use a hair dryer or electric razor when using supplemental oxygen.

WARNING: Store oxygen equipment at least five (5) feet from open flames, space heaters, large windows, or any heat source.

WARNING: Do not store a concentrator in a small enclosed space.

WARNING: Never allow the supply tube to be exposed to sharp edges, a heat source, or flame.

Stationary Systems

Stationary, or base systems provide oxygen in a fixed location and may be:

- Liquid oxygen containers with gas condensed into liquid by extreme cold.
- Concentrators with an electric motor to take nitrogen out of the air, concentrating oxygen to between 94% and 98%.
- H, S, or M60 cylinders: large tanks containing oxygen under high pressure usually used as a backup and rarely as a base system for daily use.

Liquid Oxygen

Liquid oxygen systems have a large reservoir filled by an oxygen supplier once or twice a month or as needed. These systems do not require electricity, have very few moving parts, don't usually break down, and can be easily used to fill smaller portable systems with a direct connection between the reservoir and the portable. Liquid oxygen is extremely cold and can damage your skin if spilled.

WARNING: Never have an open flame or smoking around liquid oxygen.

Compressed gas has weight. The weight of the cylinder depends partly on the amount of the compressed contents. A typical liquid-oxygen reservoir weighs about 124 pounds when filled, contains about 31 liters or 73 pounds of liquid oxygen. This amount of liquid oxygen is equivalent to 24,950 liters in gas form. Used at two liters per minute, it will last about 208 hours or eight days of use. As liquid oxygen constantly turns to gas and some oxygen must be released from the storing container to avoid excessive pressure, the container needs to be used before it bubbles away, usually within about 30 days.

Because liquid oxygen systems continually lose oxygen, even when not in use, they are appropriate for regular use at home or to fill portable systems, but are not good for emergency backup.

A small portable system with a conservation device, filled from the base reservoir could provide 20 or more trips of five to seven hours each, away from the stationary liquid oxygen before refilling the base reservoir. This means that a single fill-up each month can support a fairly active life style.

Concentrators

Oxygen concentrators are often used in the home and are probably the most economical source of supplemental oxygen. An oxygen concentrator passes room air through a powder to separate oxygen from nitrogen. The oxygen is concentrated and delivered while the nitrogen is periodically released back into the air. Concentrators are fairly small, weighing about 50-70 pounds, and need an electrical source (in North America, 110-120 volts AC). A backup oxygen supply system must be available during electrical failure.

Figure 20   Portable liquid oxygen

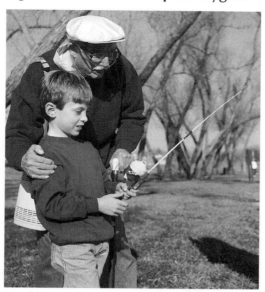

Portable liquid oxygen—here with the Nellcor Puritan Bennett Companion™ 550, which incorporates a pneumatic-demand conserving device for economy and longer use—can support an active life style.

Although older models are rather noisy, newer models are much quieter.

You need a long supply tube, up to 50 feet, and care with keeping it from tangling in furniture, people and pets—and away from sources of heat or flame.

Concentrators need routine maintenance: inspections, filter changes, and oxygen analysis. An *oxygen concentration indicator* (OCI) is now provided as an option for most oxygen concentrators, to measure the oxygen level provided by the concentrator. If the reading falls below the necessary level, an alarm is triggered. You then need to have the machine serviced. This is a valuable safety device to assure you get the correct oxygen supply. With an OCI, a phone modem may be added so that the supplier can periodically phone and connect to the concentrator to diagnose problems or confirm that all is well. This saves time for both you and the supplier while ensuring quality performance of the equipment.

Concentrators that refill portable tanks

Concentrators have often been supplied for those with COPD who are not very active and not prescribed a portable system. Some new oxygen concentrators can fill small cylinders at home, providing oxygen portability for more-active people. This type of concentrator compresses oxygen to both fill a portable cylinder and provide oxygen for breathing, both at the same time.

The first system to reach the market is the CHAD Therapeutics, Oxylite™ system. The TotalO2™ system includes concentrator, portable cylinder, and electronic conservation device. The concentrator is capable of delivering up to three liters per minute, has a sensor and alarm system with automatic shutoff in the event of system failure. The portable B/M6 unit weighs about five pounds, holds 164 liters of oxygen, and can provide eight to ten hours of use with a conserving device, at two liters per minute. The conservation device administers oxygen during the first third of inspiration, a very high level of conservation.

But at flow rates higher than four liters per minute you may need uninterrupted flow. There are three tank sizes: 40 liters, 164 liters, and a "C" size which is considerably larger. You will need backup oxygen in case of system failure or power failure.

Another concentrator which can also fill portable cylinders is the Invacare Corp, Venture™ HomeFill™ device.

Figure 21   Oxygen concentrator that refills portable cylinders

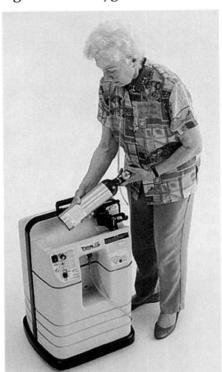

CHAD Therapeutics, Oxylite™ system. The TotalO2™ system includes the concentrator, the ability to refill the portable cylinder, and an electronic conservation device.

There are advantages to using a two-function concentrator. You have both a stationary and a portable system. With as much portable oxygen as you need, you are not dependent on a stationary supply nor on deliveries of refills.

A drawback is that the cost of oxygen is shifted to you. Instead of receiving liquid or compressed oxygen paid for by insurance, you pay for oxygen in your electrical bills for the concentrator.

Backup Systems

You may need a backup supply of oxygen as a protection against emergencies, such as loss of power to a base concentrator, the failure of a concentrator, or severe weather that might delay scheduled deliveries of compressed or liquid oxygen.

Backup systems can be either large or small, depending on your needs and location. Consider conditions where you live that could make it difficult to receive refills in an emergency, such as power outage, hurricane, ice and other storms, and flooding.

H, S, and M60 Cylinders

H, S, and M60 cylinders are large, heavy, metal tanks containing oxygen under high pressure, usually used as backup for powered systems. They do not last long enough for anyone who needs continuous oxygen, so are used as backup for a concentrator, particularly in remote areas far from a supplier. Due to their bulkiness and weight, they are hard to move, and must be secured so they can't fall over. They are usually placed on carts or cylinder stands.

Portable Systems

Portable systems provide for mobility at home, at work, and while traveling. When combined with oxygen-conserving devices they provide a surprisingly long supply in a lightweight and convenient package. They also act as backup systems for some rural people, until a supplier can restore the stationary system. Portable systems may be:

- filled from a stationary liquid oxygen container
- filled from a concentrator
- filled and delivered by the home care provider
- portable concentrators run from a car battery or other low-voltage source and are good in motor homes.

Manufacturers and rental companies recommend keeping two to three portable cylinders on hand. At a rate of two liters per minute, without a conserving device, some tanks used for backup or portability would supply:

- E cylinder (up to five hours)
- D cylinder (up to three hours)
- M9 cylinder (up to two hours)
- M6 cylinder (up to one hour).

These times can be extended by using a conserving device.

Larger tanks can be pulled on a cart or mounted in a vehicle. Smaller ones can be carried in a back or shoulder pack.

E Cylinders

E cylinders are commonly used as backup for concentrators. They weigh about 20 pounds, and can be moved on a small wheeled cart. They are fitted with a regulator to adjust flow, but usually last only a few hours, even at a rate as low as two liters per minute. They are not suitable for long-term use, and for daily use, as a sole source of oxygen, they are prohibitively expensive. E cylinders are used by airlines for passengers needing continuous oxygen while traveling. An oxygen-saving device extends the oxygen flow, even doubling it.

In the past few years, newer versions of the old heavy steel E cylinder have been developed:

- An aluminum version is much lighter and easy to carry.
- A lightweight steel tank weighs about the same as the aluminum cylinder.
- A composite tank is even lighter than the others, but more expensive.

Figure 22   E cylinders provide a backup or portable oxygen source

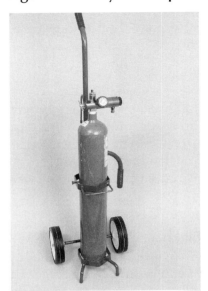

E cylinders are commonly used as backup for concentrators. They weigh between 15 and 20 pounds, and can be moved on a small wheeled cart.

Both steel and composite tanks hold a little more oxygen than the aluminum.

Portable Strollers

A portable stroller holds 7 hours of liquid O_2 at 2 l.p.m. and may be carried by a shoulder strap or wheeled on a cart.

Very Small Portable Containers

The newer, very-small portable containers are smaller and lighter-weight than E cylinders. These new containers can be filled from a large liquid oxygen tank, filled from a concentrator, or refilled by the home care provider. However, these containers have a limited capacity and are more cost effective when used with an oxygen-conserving device such as an electronic demand valve or a conserving cannula. As these cylinders are carried in a shoulder bag or back pack that looks like a black camera bag, they are less noticeable than the larger E cylinder. For active people, they are an excellent choice.

These smaller containers come in a variety of sizes, weights, and carrying options, so the size that is best for you is determined by flow rate, length of time away from source, type of cannula or oxygen-saving device, weight you can carry, and personal preference. Whether they contain compressed or liquid oxygen, they all weigh around five pounds empty. Which ones you use may also depend on the conserving device that must be used with each type of very small portable container.

Most of the operating costs of these systems come from the time it takes to refill, not the cost of the oxygen itself. A refill costs from eight to fifteen dollars per container, unless you have a concentrator that can refill smaller tanks.

Portable Concentrators

Portable concentrators run on 110/220 VAC or a 12 volt car battery. They weigh about half as much as stationary oxygen concentrators. You may be able to rent or lease the equipment, but contact the supplier well before your trip.

Figure 23 Portable stroller for oxygen

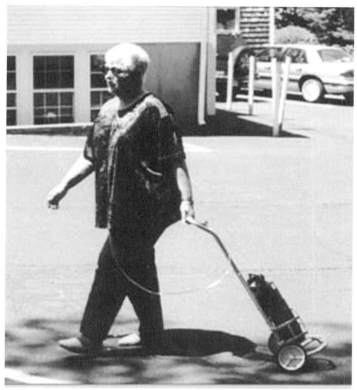

You can go about your business for many hours, assured of oxygen by your liquid portable stroller. © 1998 Frank Bumpus

Figure 24 Very small portable container and carrying case

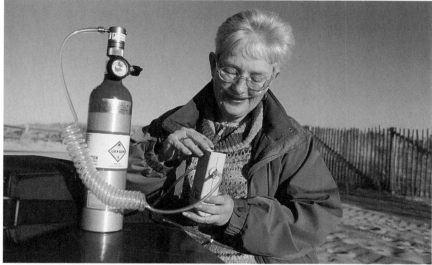

Small, lightweight oxygen containers with compressed gas can be combined with an oxygen-conserving device such as an electronic demand valve. This Oxylite™ system with a pulsed-oxygen valve easily adjusts to your varying activity needs.

Combining Storage Systems

A combination of storage systems is often used to get the most economical oxygen supply, while promoting an active life style. It is important to realize that Medicare in the United States reimburses for a portable system only if it is needed for mobility within your home, not just for away-from-home activities.

Manufacturers and rental companies recommend that two to three lightweight cylinders or containers be used with the home or base concentrator systems to provide an adequate portable oxygen source. As different flow rates change the total time any cylinder can be used, using an oxygen saving device will give more time.

Liquid systems are commonly provided with a portable backpack or walker. Usually weighing between five and a half, and eight pounds, they can be carried over the shoulder or pulled on a cart. See *Portable liquid oxygen* on page 89 and *Portable stroller for oxygen* on page 93.

Discuss advantages and disadvantages of each system with your doctor. You may wish to buy your own system rather than renting or leasing. Explore this possibility with several reputable vendors in your area and decide for yourself. Weigh the cost for each method or combination of methods, the length of a lease and comfort of the device, and do not be afraid to negotiate for the best possible deal to meet your special needs.

Figure 25   Combinations of oxygen systems

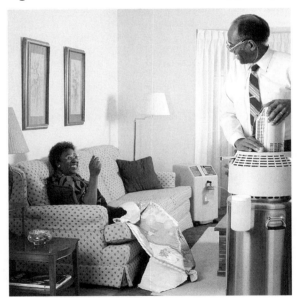

You can select a combination of oxygen systems to support your life style. Three units made by Mallinckrodt Nellcor Puritan Bennett include the Companion™ C41, a stationary system holding 73 pounds of liquid oxygen, which can be used to refill the Companion™ 550 portable liquid oxygen system. In the background is the Companion 590™ oxygen concentrator.

Support for mobility

People who have been prescribed supplemental oxygen currently have two basic choices of oxygen service. They can select, or the oxygen provider can select, an electric concentrator, which plugs into an electrical outlet and generates oxygen from room air, or they can have liquid oxygen service, which is costlier and more labor intensive for home/health care companies to provide, but which allows for greater mobility by the patient. People who are active, certainly those who continue to work outside of the home, generally prefer an oxygen system that enables them to fill a portable unit from a large stationary tank at home. Until very recently, only liquid oxygen was suitable to provide this convenience and support for mobility.

We now have a choice of small, lightweight portable systems, either those based on liquid oxygen or the new concentrators that refill portable tanks—either can allow people with COPD to maintain their social activity.

From a user's experience, consider:

Oxygen concentrators are, unfortunately, frequently left unchecked and unserviced by some home/health care companies. They must be checked periodically for oxygen output and accuracy of liter flow. Filters need cleaning.

In case of power failure, electric concentrators need to be backed up by one or more compressed-gas cylinders. Your electric bill will increase if you run a concentrator. In some parts of the United States, depending on rates, expect an increase of $60 or more per month.

Liquid oxygen systems are great for people who continue to work outside the home, or who are striving to maintain a highly active lifestyle. Stationary liquid tanks, with portable tanks that can be filled from the larger unit, provide maximum mobility and flexibility for an active person. Your medical equipment dealer will need to visit at least once a month to supply liquid oxygen.

A filled liquid portable unit may be carried on the shoulder from a strap, or pulled on a little wheeled cart. Long shopping trips will make you glad you opted for the cart.

The new concentrator systems capable of filling high-pressure gaseous oxygen tanks may prove to be equally or even more effective to support an active lifestyle.

It is important to use the small, lightweight containers with either type of portable system. I could not physically manage the heavy E-tank cylinders that may be provided by some dealers when people using electric concentrators wish to leave home for awhile. E-cylinders are just too heavy for me to lift in and out of my car. Also, a modern portable system will hold seven or more hours of oxygen, while the smaller D-cylinder or M6 only hold about one and a half hours worth, unless oxygen-saver devices are used. I would need dozens of the small cylinders just to get me back and forth between work and home.

In my case, a light, portable system allows me to continue working and supporting myself, rather than falling back on a disability income.   *JVT*

Oxygen Breathing Equipment

Nasal Cannulas

The nasal cannula is the most common form of oxygen delivery. They are inexpensive, relatively comfortable, provide a great deal of flexibility, and allow you to pursue daily activities. You can talk, eat and cough while wearing them.

Figure 26   Nasal cannula for delivering oxygen

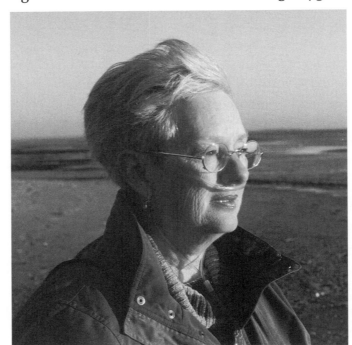

Wearing an oxygen cannula on the face does not interfere with talking and eating.

A nasal cannula has two small prongs in the nose attached to a tube coming from an oxygen source. Two to six liters of oxygen per minute can be administered, but consistent use of more than three liters per minute may dry the lining of the nose and lead to sinusitis. Bubbling the oxygen through a humidifier before delivery at the nose moistens the gas. At low oxygen flow rates of one or two liters per minute, or with a conserving cannula, it may not be necessary to moisten the gas.

I am on two liters per minute and benefit from using a humidifier on both my home and office stationary tanks.   *JVT*

A nasal cannula may also produce some irritation around the ears. Padding over the ear with a soft cloth or a wrapping around the tubing at the ear may help correct this. There is also a adjustable head band which may be used to hold the cannula and take pressure off the ears. This can be easily made with a strip of cloth with Velcro which is attached to the cannula over the temple area and sits on the crown of the head or supports the cannula by pulling to the back of the head. This simple device should be located where the point of irritation is for each patient.

Oxygen Conserving Equipment

Oxygen flow can be significantly reduced by using an *oxygen-conserving device* to reduce flow while maintaining the same level of oxygen delivery. Depending on the device, the flow of oxygen stops momentarily, while you exhale, during part of your inhalation, or both.

Oxygen-conserving devices can lengthen use of a tank by up to eight times. This is because the oxygen that would normally be wasted while you exhale, is saved. However savings depend on how you use the device, the type of device, and the rate of oxygen flow.

An oxygen-conserving device allows you to carry a lighter tank or to remain mobile longer.

Example

A portable liquid oxygen system that weighs about five pounds can support a flow rate of two liters per minute for about four and a half hours. With a conserving device the same tank could provide up to eight and a half hours of use.

Conserving Nasal Cannula

Since a standard nasal cannula delivers continuous oxygen, it wastes the oxygen delivered during exhalation and is expensive. Nasal cannulas which conserve oxygen while maintaining delivery use a reduced flow rate because they store oxygen in a small reservoir during exhalation. At the beginning of inhalation the storage reservoir releases its stored oxygen so that oxygen normally lost during exhalation is saved and used during the next breath.

Studies have demonstrated that savings can range from 40% to 70%. This means that you can receive the same amount of oxygen in your lungs at a flow rate of one liter per minute as you do with two to three liters per minute using an ordinary nasal cannula. As oxygen-conserving cannulas allow lower flows, they are also less likely to dry the nose lining.

Ask your doctor or therapist about these devices.

Pulsed Oxygen Delivery with Nasal Cannula

Electronic devices to save oxygen have been developed to electronically sense the start of inhalation and deliver a prescribed amount of oxygen, with every breath, or with every second or third breath. These devices use only a fraction of the oxygen delivered by an ordinary cannula without sensing equipment. They allow you to remain on a portable much longer than using a traditional, non-pulsed system: as much as two to seven or eight times longer, depending on the device and how you use it.

Similar benefits are possible using devices which sense air-pressure changes during breathing, rather than sensing electronically.

The amount of oxygen a person needs to receive per minute can be set by a battery-powered device, and based on the number of breaths a person takes. The heart of the system is a small control unit between the oxygen canister and the nasal cannula. These systems have alarms for system malfunctions or low battery.

There are several types of pulsed-oxygen delivery systems. Although you will probably quickly adjust to and ignore the sound of the valve, there may be some business and social situations where noise is distracting. If this is important to

Figure 27   Oxygen-conserving nasal cannula

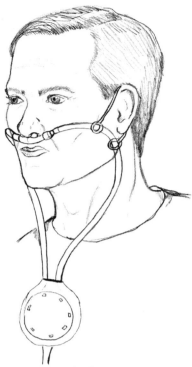

Nasal cannulas which conserve oxygen while maintaining delivery use a reduced flow rate because they store oxygen in a small reservoir during exhalation. At the beginning of inhalation the Oxymizer™ storage reservoir releases its stored oxygen so that oxygen normally lost during exhalation is saved and used during the next breath.

Figure 28   Pulsed oxygen delivery with nasal cannula

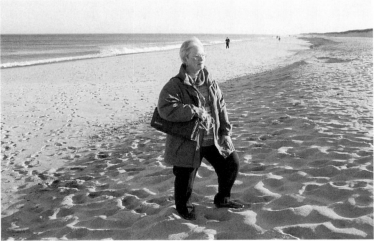

Pulsed-oxygen delivery systems like the Oxylite™ are lightweight and portable, allowing you great freedom for many hours, wherever you want to go.

you, select a unit that can be set for constant flow during times when the sound of operation could be a problem. You will have to remember to adjust your extended oxygen-use schedule.

Fixed-pulse device: a sensor detects inhalation and delivers a burst of oxygen, usually for a fixed length of time that is less than a full inspiration. The device may be set to deliver oxygen at various rates and with each breath, or it may be set to skip one or more breaths.

Demand-pulse device: can deliver oxygen during the whole inspiration or during part of the cycle and is able to adapt to changing demands.

Variable-demand device: continuously monitors and measures the rate and length of each breath and adjusts oxygen delivered.

Selecting a Conserving Device

The main advantage of a conserving device is to give you as many hours of use as possible, by reducing the size and weight of your portable oxygen support system, while providing a normal level of blood oxygen. As prescriptions for oxygen are usually for continuous flow, your prescription needs to be revised or adapted for use with a conserving device. Work with your respiratory therapist and physician to consider your personal life-style as well as oxygen requirements.

Whatever system you consider needs to be tested when you are active as well as while you are at rest, to see if your blood oxygen can be maintained at a good level. The levels will be recorded and prescribed by your doctor for your various levels of activity.

The system needs a fail-safe to revert to full oxygen flow in several circumstances: in the absence of a breath, if the breathing rate goes very high, or if the device fails. You will need to learn what setting to use in each situation and how long your oxygen canister can support you at each level.

Alternatives For Delivering Oxygen

Face Masks

For people with very low oxygen levels, using a tightly fitting face mask is one way to deliver a lot of oxygen. For people with COPD, the use of such high concentrations may decrease the level of breathing and be dangerous.

Face masks for oxygen delivery are not often used outside a hospital. For people who are very ill, a type of mask called the Venti-mask is used to deliver exact amounts of oxygen. These masks provide a constant, predetermined oxygen concentration, with close regulation, to minimize the chance that a person decreases breathing due to too much oxygen.

Masks are not as well tolerated as nasal cannulas. Particularly for people who are already short of breath, they may cause a panicky feeling of smothering. Masks make it hard to eat, talk, and spit. They are rarely a successful long-term solution.

Transtracheal Oxygen Delivery (TTO)

Transtracheal oxygen delivery is efficient, cosmetically more acceptable for some people, promotes continuous use of oxygen, and reduces breathlessness during eating. For example, a person needing two liters per minute with a regular cannula may need only one liter per minute with a *transtracheal catheter*. This lengthens the amount of time for one E cylinder from five hours to ten. The transtracheal catheter can also be combined with an electronic pulsed-oxygen device for greater efficiency. The system requires a surgical procedure with its potential problems, the most common, spasms of cough during and after catheter placement. Probably for these reasons, the catheter has never been widely used. There are standard methods for inserting a catheter (small tube) through the skin at the front of the neck into the windpipe to enable the direct delivery of oxygen into the trachea. A needle is inserted through the cricothyroid mem-

Figure 29   Transtracheal oxygen delivery

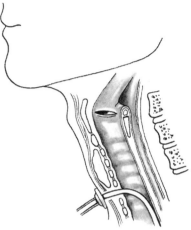

Transtracheal oxygen delivery is efficient, cosmetically more acceptable for some people, promotes continuous use of oxygen, and reduces breathlessness during eating. The surgical procedure to introduce a catheter is not complicated.

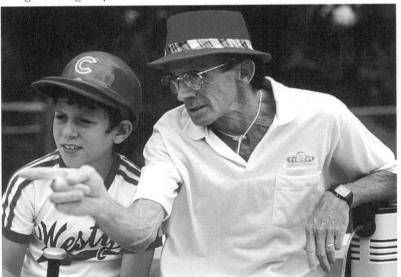

Using the SCOOP® Oxygen Therapy system for transtracheal oxygen delivery.

brane. Then a catheter is introduced through the needle and remains in place after the needle is withdrawn. The oxygen source is connected to the small tube. In order to prevent infection, the catheter needs attention and cleaning on a daily basis.

Costs of Systems

The cost of renting, leasing or buying equipment varies from region to region, and country to country. It is important to discuss the advantages and disadvantages of systems with your doctor and oxygen-supply company. Costs and services will also differ between oxygen-supply companies. Explore possibilities and select the one that meets your needs. We recommend that you rent a system you are considering buying, for a month or longer, to make sure it meets your needs.

Most vendors offer maintenance agreements for the equipment they supply or alternative service agreements. Check that the maintenance agreement:

• Is affordable
• Covers parts and repairs
• Lends equipment when yours is being serviced
• States clearly all conditions of the contract.

When selecting a supplier, if the company is accredited by the Joint Commission for Accreditation of Health Care Organizations (JCAHO), you will have assurance the products and supplies will meet national standards.

Because of competition, equipment costs have come down, so the biggest difference among vendors is in service. Ask several companies to outline their services and costs. Ask if they have respiratory therapists on staff. Ask for a written bid.

Suppliers in some areas will provide liquid oxygen for active people through Medicare if requested and prescribed by the physician. Reimbursement amounts and contracts are not uniform in different areas of the United States and elsewhere. Private insurance may reimburse equipment costs. Talk to your doctor and the medical supplier.

Base concentrator systems capable of supplying your portable tank cost about twice as much as a simple concentrator, for the initial setup. The same problems occur with supplier reimbursement.

Liquid oxygen home based systems capable of supplying your portable tanks cost more than an ordinary system. The same reimbursement problems experienced with home concentrator systems occur. Talk to your doctor and the medical supplier.

United States Medicare and Other Insurance

Medicare in the US will only pay a standard rental to the supply company regardless of the type of system. The oxygen-supply company will lose money if it provides you with a more expensive system which will not be reimbursed. Your doctor may prescribe a specific type of system for you, however the supply company may find it difficult or impossible to supply that system without adequate reimbursement. The supply company may prefer to use the least expensive system. This must be resolved by negotiation between your doctor and the supply company. The result may be that even though your doctor prescribes a more expensive system, you may not get it, since Medicare does not allow you to pay extra to the provider company.

A person on Medicare may buy a system outright, but it is expensive and also requires upkeep. With other insurance such as HMO contracts, you may have to pay the difference between the systems covered and a system you prefer.

U.S. Medicare currently covers some of the cost of oxygen for those who need it continuously, but not only for use during exercise and not only for portable systems.

Liquid oxygen systems need more service from home/health care providers, and are not fully reimbursed. With 25% cuts to reimbursement for oxygen implemented in January of 1998, many health care companies are attempting to remove liquid oxygen from some people. By law, however, the oxygen provider cannot change the method of oxygen delivery prescribed by the doctor. Another 5% cut in U.S. Medicare reimbursement took place in January, 1999. *JVT*

Issues of Limited Health Care Resources in the United States

In the United States, we live in a time of drastically changing health care. Hospitals and clinics are fighting to stay in business. In most cases, they are being run by business people, not by medical personnel. Many of them have taken serious steps to economize, including downsizing and eliminating many areas of medical treatment that were provided before today's economic pressures.

As a result, there seem to be fewer doctors on call for Emergency Room service, fewer nurses available throughout hospitals and doctor's offices, fewer hospital-sponsored support groups and health lectures offered. And, worst of all, it seems that insurance companies are calling too many of the shots relating to patient care, treatment, tests and coverage for services. They are particularly hard-nosed about treatments and surgeries they deem to be experimental, and therefore not covered.

The cycle is seemingly endless. Medicare and private insurance companies pay private practice physicians less for their services than before. Doctors then have to see more patients in order to make up for the drop in their income. They still have nurses, physician's assistants, secretarial, billing, and bookkeeping personnel, equipment constantly in need of upgrade, malpractice insurance, and many other operating expenses to cover, plus their own salaries. So these circumstances have created the ten-minute-office-visit syndrome.

During 1997 the United States Congress passed, and President Clinton signed into action, an across-the-board cut of 25% for Medicare coverage for oxygen reimbursements. These measures were effective January 1, 1998. Another 5% cut was added to the federal budget's Medicare program in 1999, totaling 30% reduction in oxygen reimbursements and coverage by Medicare. Private insurers follow Medicare guidelines. So these cuts will be felt most by elderly and ill people, particularly COPD patients. Additional cuts may be enacted based on information from the United States Government Accounting Office (GAO). These cuts are being implemented to control the outlay of Medicare dollars now and in the future.

For example, the companies that provide oxygen equipment and service claim that they cannot withstand 25 and 30% cuts in their income. Many of them further claim that they were losing money even before such drastic cuts were implemented. As a result, there is much talk within the home/health care industry of entire types of service being eliminated, such as liquid oxygen.

Oxygen concentrators (see *Concentrators* on page 88) are often used as an economical source of supplemental oxygen. A new system which allows for filling portable containers from a concentrator is now available. It will probably replace the liquid systems, especially when used with an oxygen-saving delivery system. But the patient must check to be sure that such equipment is available and is covered by insurance. See *Oxygen Storage Systems* on page 87 and *Combining Storage Systems* on page 94.

Actions are being taken by support groups and individuals all over the United States to bring the issue to the attention of legislators who can help us by line-item treatment of oxygen service reimbursement. Get involved in the fight to roll back the cuts for this lifeline for those with COPD. Write letters, make phone calls, apply pressure any way you can. We need your help. *JVT*

Publisher's Note: TransTracheal Systems has commented on the text under **(Transtracheal Oxygen Delivery (TTO), on page 99)** and the illustration **(Transtracheal oxygen delivery, on page 100)**. They have advised the publisher that TransTracheal Systems currently recommends a different procedure than the one described and pictured here. They claim that their recommended procedures for the placement of the transtracheal oxygen catheter cause less problems than here suggested in terms of hoarseness or coughing. Therefore, as with all information in this book, we recommend that readers considering transtracheal oxygen delivery should consult with their own physician regarding treatments including decisions on procedures and possible outcomes.

6 Smoking

Why Quit?

Stopping smoking is probably the most important step that you can take to improve your health, and it is never too late to quit. Smoking is linked to premature heart and blood vessel disease, cancer, and lung disease. Long term smoking causes changes in the lung that are permanent and will not completely reverse because you stop smoking. But no matter how long you've smoked, stopping has positive effects.

What Happens When You Stop Smoking

For most who cough up sputum daily, stopping smoking will decrease the frequency of coughing and will cut down the amount of phlegm which has to be coughed up daily. Clearing out the remaining phlegm is easier when there is no more smoke around to damage the cilia that help the lungs to move phlegm out.

Production of phlegm and the need to cough it up may actually increase for the first two to three weeks after you stop smoking as the lung tries to recover and to clean out pollutants. After that, phlegm should decrease, and you should feel much better.

Frequency of respiratory infections and allergies should also decrease when you quit.

Cigarette smoke does damage as a direct irritant of the bronchial tubes and can increase attacks of wheezing, leading to increased shortness of breath and exacerbations of COPD. This also improves when you stop smoking, and as the wheezing decreases, breathing may improve.

Smoke also damages the lining of the nose and the sinuses. Continuous nasal drainage, postnasal drip, persistent or recurrent sinusitis, are all caused or worsened by smoking. Nasal and sinus problems may make the lung problems worse as mucus drains down the back of the throat, causes cough and aggravates wheezing. What smokers often call allergies or colds are actually irritations due to smoke exposure. This is an area where a large improvement may occur after you quit.

A main pollutant in cigarette smoke is carbon monoxide (CO). It is different from carbon dioxide (CO_2) produced by your body. When carbon monoxide enters the blood, it competes with oxygen preventing oxygen molecules from entering the blood. The more you smoke the higher the carbon monoxide level in your blood and the lower the amount of available oxygen. This is what kills people when they inhale smoke in a fire. They suffocate.

Smokers frequently have seven to eleven percent of their hemoglobin attached to carbon monoxide. Death in fire by suffocation occurs when carbon monoxide is attached to over 40% of the hemoglobin. There isn't enough oxygen for the cells to work, particularly the heart, so smokers have more heart attacks and irregular heart beats than non-smokers. In fact, your risk of sudden death or of a heart attack drops within the first *day* after you quit smoking.

Automobile fumes also carry large amounts of carbon monoxide. Leaky exhaust systems in cars need to be promptly repaired, as these fumes can leak into cars and cause major problems, and not only for people with COPD.

Many people do not realize that smoking causes damage to the blood vessels. This is a major risk for heart disease and strokes. Particularly in men, smoking prevents normal sexual performance. The blood vessels may not fill normally and since an erection requires the blood vessels in the penis to fill with extra blood, a normal erection may not occur.

After You Stop

One complaint heard from recent ex-smokers is, "I stopped smoking and I'm not breathing any easier." The positive effects of quitting take time to develop, possibly months, and some symptoms may get better while others don't. However, the benefits for lung function are clear.

Lung function declines gradually over a period of years in a normally aging person, and contrasts with lung function in those with COPD. The normal person, or the smoker who is not susceptible to COPD, is not disabled or killed by the loss of lung capacity. The person who has COPD and continues to smoke loses lung capacity so quickly that they may be disabled when they have only 25 percent of lung capacity remaining, or die when the capacity goes down to about 10 percent. The drop off in lung function with aging is much higher and occurs sooner in COPD with those who still smoke. Ex-smokers may experience a normal drop off rate after a while. Unfortunately, since with COPD there is already damage, lungs cannot return to normal. The length of time before disability and death is definitely better for those who stop smoking than for those who continue. (See *Stop smoking to reduce the loss of lung function* on page 107).

The figure shows what happens to the average person, not what happens to a particular individual. You may react better or worse than the average. For example, a group with an average age of 50 years might be made up entirely of persons between 40 and 60 years old. On the other hand, people 10 and 90 years old may be in the group. Either way, the average or mean age is 50.

Figure 30   Stop smoking to reduce the loss of lung function

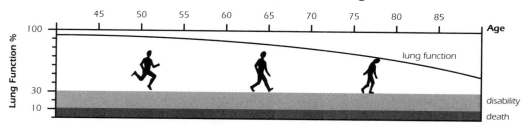

Lung function is gradually lost as the healthy, non-smoking person ages, but will probably not become a cause of disability or death.

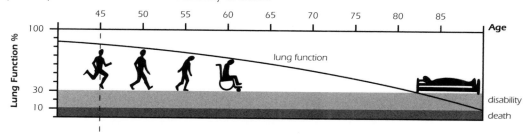

Stopped smoking at age 45

A susceptible smoker experiences a more rapid rate of decline. Smoking progressively reduces lung capacity, and this reduction is added to the normal loss of aging. Thus if you are susceptible and continue to smoke, you hasten the approach of disability and death. Disability happens when your lung function reaches about 30 percent and death happens when your lung function is about 10 percent of normal. If you stop smoking at age 45, the lung function tends to be lost at the slower rate of decline of the normal person, although the damage that has been done remains.

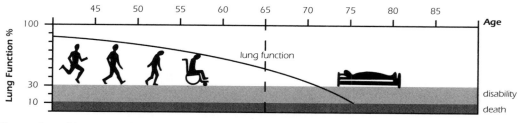

Stopped smoking at age 65

The longer a person continues to smoke, the greater the damage, however even stopping at 65 provides the potential of survival benefit and better quality of life. The sooner you stop, the better your chance to retain lung function.

Other factors related to cigarette smoking also improve when you stop, though they may take longer. For example, your risk for lung and other cancers gradually decreases, but it takes over 10 years before you become similar to a non-smoker in risk. As people with COPD are at greater risk of lung cancer than other smokers, any decrease in risk is a benefit.

Cigarette smoking increases the risk of stroke, even before age 65, during your most productive years. Stopping smoking reduces this risk.

Financial benefits of stopping smoking are significant. The cost of one pack of cigarettes in 1998 ranged from $1.50 to $2.00 in the United States. This amounts to $45-$60 a month at one pack a day. The U.S. Congress wants to increase the tax on each packet of cigarettes by $.75 to $1.00. Buying cigarettes is a large and growing burden for an average household.

Weight Gain

When you quit smoking, you may gain weight. Average weight gain is only about five to seven pounds, although this can vary, but less than one smoker out of thirty who quits gains more than 20 pounds. Two main reasons for the weight gain are: your taste improves, and your metabolism changes.

Cigarette smoke damages the taste buds just as it damages other parts of the body. Nicotine speeds up your metabolism so that as a smoker you can eat more calories without weight gain. When you quit, as the taste buds recover, foods taste better and your appetite improves. If you use nicotine replacement to help quit, you may put off metabolism change for a time. If you are prone to weight gain, or are already overweight, watch what you eat after you give up cigarettes. Eat more fruits and vegetables. Avoid fatty foods and foods with a lot of calories. Don't snack right before bed. Drink lots of water, and increase your level of exercise.

Psychological Effects

Smokers almost universally feel guilty about continuing to smoke. At the same time, they feel defeated because they are not strong enough to "kick the habit." Often people feel much better psychologically after they quit, and have more energy. Successfully giving up cigarettes leads to feelings of power over your own body and triumph because you are strong enough to quit. In fact, ex-smokers sometimes become almost rabid about the bad habits of continuing smokers. They have been known to sneer and make comments about lack of willpower.

Quitting

Difficulty of Quitting an Addiction

Any doctor who listens to patient after patient say "I know that these cigarettes are killing me but I can't quit" recognizes addiction. If you are having a great deal of difficulty quitting, there are reasons:

- Nicotine is an addicting substance. In spite of what the tobacco companies say, smoking meets the World Health Organization definition for addiction and dependence. This definition states that drug dependence is a psychological and sometimes physical state which results from interaction between the body and a drug. There is a compulsion to take in the drug on a continuous or periodic basis to experience the psychic effects or to avoid discomfort from not taking the drug.
- Cigarettes contain as many as 4,000 chemicals (drugs) besides nicotine. But we know more about nicotine than the others so it is the most discussed.
- Nicotine actually sets up the brain to continuously crave more nicotine. Addicted smokers may wake in the night wanting a cigarette so badly that they will stumble, coughing, through a dark house or even go to the store through a dangerous neighborhood to get one. Some patients with COPD will remove their oxygen in order to smoke, or worse, smoke through a tracheostomy, a hole in the windpipe created to help breathing in special circumstances. In spite of dirty looks, condescending comments from co-

workers, the smoker stands outside in below-freezing weather to have a cigarette. The addicted smoker is willing to risk slower professional advancement and a second class citizen status in order to smoke.

- Quitting is *not easy*! Over 75% of smokers say they would like to quit and two out of three have made at least one serious attempt to quit. Most smokers trying to quit are irritable and nervous. They may try to substitute food for the cigarette and eat constantly.

- Often smokers who try to quit experience a desire for a cigarette so intense that they have trouble concentrating on anything else. The act of smoking may be addictive as well as the nicotine. Help for these symptoms is available, however, as nicotine replacement techniques reverse most of the withdrawal symptoms.

- Nicotine replacement may not help the desire for a cigarette; this is one reason that quitting is so difficult in spite of a strong desire to stop.

- Inhaled nicotine also has positive effects. Nicotine improves performance of some tasks and increases alertness. It can cause euphoria, a feeling that everything's going well. It reduces mild depression and anxiety.

- Many people return to smoking in response to stress or conflict. It is important to recognize that these are underlying factors and deal with them openly.

- Social acceptance and peer pressure encourage smoking. The tobacco companies have taken advantage of this by targeting youngsters. They show smoking as an assertion of independence from adults, and as a factor for acceptance in a group. The tobacco companies have also aimed a huge amount of advertising at African-Americans, trying to make smoking a positive self-image factor. Unfortunately, they have been successful and there is a disproportionate number of African-American people with smoking-related disease.

Ways to Quit

In spite of these problems, some smokers do quit permanently. How do they do that?

For most folks it is not easy. Even with serious diseases related directly to cigarette smoking, people find it hard to quit. For every person who just lays down the cigarette and walks away forever, there are lots more who try and try without success.

Studies of large groups of smokers have identified four stages of quitting.

Stage 1 is *precontemplation* and includes people who have not decided to quit smoking within the next six months. These people are very unlikely to quit.

Stage 2 is *contemplation* and includes people who intend to quit within the next six months, but have not yet started to do so.

Stage 3 is *action*. Most ex-smokers come from this group.

Stage 4 is *maintenance*, after more than six months of not smoking. If you slip and start smoking again you are back to Stage 1. If you slip but intend to quit within the next month, then you're back at Stage 2.

The first group to join is Stage 2. You *must* first make up your mind that you really want to quit, then do it. If you don't really want to quit, no method will succeed.

Less than five people out of one hundred who've decided to quit can do so on the first try. Most ex-smokers make a serious effort to quit at least three to four times before they get off cigarettes for good. That is, they may stop for a while, restart, again decide to quit, then stop again. So don't get discouraged. You have a chance as long as you're in at least Stage 2.

There are many types of programs to help you stop smoking, but the simplest is your own decision to put the cigarette down and never pick up another. This is rarely successful even in people with serious health problems. If a recommendation to quit comes from the doctor, quitting levels are slightly better but still very poor. Other methods include *behavior modification*, *pharmacologic methods*, and acupuncture.

Behavior modification programs

Behavior modification can be approached in many different ways.

- One approach is to try to get you to see smoking as a very negative habit. You are urged to list all the reasons why you should quit, and list all the harm that the cigarettes are doing. Medical consequences are stressed, but also important are harmful effects on family members, particularly children, the social unacceptability and unpleasantness of smoking, and the financial costs.
- Another approach is to try to convince you of the highly positive medical and social effects of being an ex-smoker. These programs promote positive self-image, which is enhanced if the smoker actually quits.
- Most programs combine both approaches. Both approaches stress that it is possible to quit, even if you've failed before. Many techniques are included to help you realize and avoid high-risk behaviors: events where many people are smoking, drinking alcohol, smoking to relieve stress.
- It is not clear whether abrupt or gradual quitting is best. Some programs allow you to select. Some programs include negative physical stimulation with behavioral modification, to improve quit rates: rapid-smoking techniques or small electric shocks associate smoking with painful and unpleasant experiences. But these techniques have not proved particularly effective. For people with heart disease, such techniques are actually dangerous.

Pharmacologic methods

Pharmacologic methods using a variety of different drugs have been tried.

WARNING: **Important: stop smoking completely as soon as you start nicotine replacement. If you don't, you can get an overdose of nicotine, which is unpleasant or even dangerous, especially if you have heart disease.**

WARNING: **Use nicotine in any form very carefully with heart disease, especially with angina (chest pain coming from the heart) or with irregular heart beat.**

- Drugs such as *lobeline sulfate*, available without prescription, do not have improved quitting statistics.
- *Nicotine gum* and *nicotine skin patch* studies show greater success rates than placebos (substances with no effects). These medications no longer require a prescription in the United States, and are most successful when combined with behavior modification. Inhaled nicotine, requiring a prescription, is now available and may be more effective than the gum or patch.
- One problem with both nicotine-replacement methods is that you may not get enough nicotine. The intent is that enough medication is given to achieve about one-half as much nicotine in your system as you get through smoking.

This amount is felt to be enough to prevent withdrawal symptoms, but not enough to totally replace the nicotine from cigarettes, avoiding dependence on the new source of nicotine. The medication is used at this level for several months, then gradually tapered and discontinued. Unfortunately, no allowance is made for body size or the amount smoked.

- Instructions with the gum, "Use as directed," are not helpful. Under-dosage often leads to anxiety, nervousness, tremor and depression. Another problem is that the level of nicotine which gets into your system depends entirely on how fast you chew the gum. Rapid chewing can produce nausea, dizziness, and palpitations due to a high nicotine level.

- With the patch this is less often a problem, although excessive nicotine can be absorbed through the skin and cause symptoms, particularly for light smokers. Major symptoms with the patch are dizziness, insomnia and disturbing dreams.

- Only rarely has the gum or patch become addicting.

- A new medicine, bupropion HCL (Zyban®), has been helpful for many people. It doesn't contain nicotine, is in pill form, and requires a prescription. It decreases desire for a cigarette and cuts down on nervousness while you are quitting. According to a report in the *New England Journal of Medicine* (March 4, 1999, Vol 340 No.9), very good results were obtained in a controlled clinical trial. The percentages of people who continued to abstain from smoking a year after treatment were: 30 percent of those who had used sustained-release bupropion, and 35.5 percent for those who had used buproprion and the nicotine patch together—compared with 15.6 percent of those who used a placebo and 16.4 percent of those who used only the nicotine patch.

Other methods

Other methods such as acupuncture are being more widely used. Usually acupuncture is combined with counseling and hypnosis, individually or in a group. Success rates are highly variable, and these methods may be more effective when combined with the other techniques.

Advice on Quitting from the Professionals

As professionals who treat a large number of people with COPD who wish to quit smoking, we do not have any magic methods.

The decision to quit is the first step. Start by listing all the negative things about cigarettes for you personally and for your family. Then list the positive things about smoking and decide if the positives could be achieved in some way that is less destructive and expensive.

After you decide to quit, your next decision is whether to do it suddenly or gradually. If you smoke more than one and a half packages of cigarettes daily, you probably need to cut down before trying nicotine replacement therapy. The strongest patches can't replace nicotine for heavy smokers.

If you are going to cut down and gradually stop, make it easier on yourself by making it less convenient to have a cigarette:

- Don't keep the cigarettes in your pocket or purse, keep them on the top back shelf of the pantry.

- Don't sit around the table talking after meals, go for a walk or to a movie.

- Don't go to the corner bar for drinks with the boys, or the girls. Avoid this for at least several months unless they are all non-smokers. Alcohol seems to make nicotine craving worse.
- Drink less coffee or stop drinking it altogether. Caffeine can aggravate your desire for a cigarette. Switch to juice or milk or even hot water.
- Carry a little book around with you and write about every cigarette you smoke and why you had to have it.
- Avoid smokers. If you are going to quit suddenly, it is even more important to avoid surrounding yourself with smokers. "Avoid the occasions of sin" as the preachers used to say.
- It may be particularly difficult to quit smoking when others in your house, particularly your spouse, continue to do so. Discuss it with them. They may wish to try to quit with you. At the very least, ask them to only smoke outside. Ask your doctor to talk to them about the need for you to avoid smoke, if they are still hesitant.
- Think of yourself as an ex-smoker, free from the need to spend money you can not afford on junk you don't need.
- Add up the extra money you will have in a month if you don't smoke, and decide how you will spend this windfall.
- Savor the pleasure you'll get from reducing the income of your already well-off doctor, or worse, the tobacco company executive.
- Put a sign on your door forbidding other family members or friends to smoke in your home. Don't hesitate. Tell these people how important it is for you to quit. Most will be happy to help you.
- Think how triumphant you will feel when you kick the habit.

Nicotine Replacement

If your doctor prescribes nicotine replacement therapy, be sure you use a large enough amount for a long enough time to do the job.

The advantage to the patch is that you don't have to continue using it forever and it is less harmful than smoking. With the patch, most studies were done using the highest milligram dose for six or twelve weeks, then continuing with mid-level and low-level doses for at least another four to twelve weeks. This is a total of at least three to four months. In the United States, the patches cost about $3.00 each in 1998, so you will have to spend between $270.00 to $360.00 for the average course. At one pack a day of cigarettes for one year, you would spend $547.50, if each pack costs $1.50.

If you use the gum, you can expect to chew twelve to sixteen pieces a day for the first several weeks. After that, you may gradually decrease the amount chewed, but you are likely to still need eight or more pieces a day at the third or fourth month. You should have the gum available for stressful situations for at least six months after you have your last cigarette.

Chew the gum slowly when starting a fresh piece. The manufacturer recommends three or four chews, then either "parking" the gum in the corner of your mouth or taking it out altogether. The longer you chew a piece, the less nicotine it has, so we recommend that you use a regular dosage of one piece per hour while you are awake when you first quit, so that the craving does not get to be too much. It is easier to prevent the craving than to treat after it starts. The cost for an average of 12 pieces a day for two months will be about $400.00.

Community Programs

If you're not successful on your own, get into a community program. There are usually low cost programs available through non-profit groups. Become a knowledgeable consumer by reading all you can about stop-smoking programs, and speaking with your doctor, pharmacist, nurse and friends about programs in the community which work. Good sources of information are the American Lung Association, The American Heart Association, The American Cancer Society, and your local hospital.

Investigate the success rate and probable cost of the program before entering.

Most important of all, if you don't succeed at first, don't give up. Quitting is hard. Like an athlete trying to set a world record, you may need to keep practicing until you are perfect. Don't be impatient with yourself, but try to understand why you haven't succeeded, make corrections, and try again.

7 Sleep and Sex

Sleep Disturbance

Sleep disturbances are very common in people with COPD. These may be due to the lung disease itself. Sometimes just lying down can increase difficulty in breathing and interfere with the process of getting oxygen into the blood. This is why many people spend the night sitting up in a recliner or on a sofa. They can't tolerate lying down.

High-quality sleep is a basic requirement of human beings. Controlled by an internal clock, we are most sleepy at night and in the early afternoon. At these times, accidents occur more frequently due to falling asleep, although the amount of sleep needed to remain alert during the day varies from person to person. If you sleep enough at night, you should not fall asleep in passive situations such as driving or reading.

Sleep loss can shorten your attention span and lengthen your reaction time. Quality sleep depends on the amount of time and the quality of your sleep, not simply being in bed.

Many things can alter sleep patterns and reduce its quality. With COPD, a significant cause of low oxygen levels is poor breathing while sleeping. In normal people, breathing is reduced in all stages of sleep compared to breathing while awake. A time during sleep when the eyes move rapidly under the closed eyelids, known as the rapid eye movement (REM) stage, is the period of sleep where the most dramatic fall in oxygen occurs, even in normal people. Everyone needs a lot of REM sleep every night, but if lung disease is present, low oxygen level during this time may waken you and cause sleep to be unrestful.

Sleep has been subdivided into five stages based on brain-wave measurements: Stages 1 to 4 and REM sleep. Good sleep needs REM sleep and some time in the other stages each night. If your oxygen level goes down too much during sleep, you waken periodically and have *fragmented sleep*. In the morning you have trouble waking up, feeling tired and unrefreshed.

Sleep may also be affected by medications used to treat COPD. For example, theophylline, a stimulant that promotes dilation of the airways is in the same class of chemicals as caffeine. You may have difficulty falling asleep and staying asleep after taking theophylline, especially in large doses. Diuretics may also compromise sleep, if you have to get up frequently to urinate. Try to avoid taking these medications before bedtime. Changes in the type of medication used or in the dosing regime may be needed, so discuss these issues with your doctor.

Sleep Apnea

People with COPD may also have sleep apnea, a common condition in which there are repeated pauses in breathing during sleep—breathing stops for many seconds. Sleep apnea results in daytime sleepiness, sometimes so severe that people fall asleep in dangerous situations while driving or ironing, or in embarrassing ones such as talking.

There are three types of sleep apnea.

Obstructive sleep apnea is caused by airflow blockage in the upper back of the throat, often caused by the relaxation of the upper airway or by the tongue. Symptoms may include loud snoring, repeated pauses in breathing lasting longer than 10 seconds, and periodic gasps when the person awakens partially and resumes breathing. Snoring and *hypopnea* (a reduction in airflow) can also affect sleep quality.

During the day, while awake, your brain keeps the upper airway from relaxing too much. At night, the upper airway relaxes, and the tongue may fall back and block the airway. When this happens, you struggle to breathe but no air is able to get in. After a time, low oxygen or the struggle itself wakes you. Then the muscles again open the airway and the tongue is removed from the airway and breathing resumes. It is easy to see why you are tired the next day. You are struggling to breathe during much of the night, sleep has been fragmented, or broken into short moments and the restorative cycle of sleep can not take place.

Central apnea is the failure of the brain to signal the lungs that it is time to take a breath. This is less often the sole cause of sleep disturbance in people with COPD.

Mixed apnea consists of both a decrease in the effort to breath and airway obstruction.

In less severe cases the person may be unaware that sleep disturbances have occurred, yet will waken unrefreshed. If you complain of sleepiness or poor quality sleep, or someone has told you that you snore heavily, or have many long pauses in your breathing, ask your doctor about it. For more information on obstructive sleep apnea syndrome, read the latest edition of *Phantom of the Night*[1], a handbook for patients.

---

1. T.S. Johnson, MD, J. Halberstadt, and W. Broughton, *Phantom of the Night*, 1999

Treating Obstructive Sleep Apnea

This is a treatable condition in most people. Whatever treatment is chosen for sleep apnea, success needs to be confirmed by an overnight study. Losing weight is a practical prescription for some, made easier if apnea is first controlled with CPAP positive airway pressure (PAP). Weight loss in overweight people also provides other health benefits, and when accomplished with exercise, benefits increase dramatically. See *Losing weight* on page 148.

A custom mouthpiece (oral device or dental appliance) can be worn at night to treat mild problems with restricted airflow during sleep, and in some individuals this method has been helpful treating sleep apnea. A sleep specialist, ear-nose-throat specialist, or dentist may be able to make this mouthpiece for you. It is advisable to confirm the success of the treatment with an overnight sleep study (polysomnography) carried out by a qualified sleep disorders center.

To assure restful sleep, it is necessary to prevent apneic episodes; that is, prevent the breathing stoppage. It is also important to eliminate the fragmentation of sleep. If the reason for apnea is that the upper airway is closed off by a large tongue or by the collapse of the upper airway, air under positive pressure pushing out against the tissue can correct the problem. This is usually applied by a mask over the nose, worn all night to increase the air pressure in the upper airway. The pressures needed to keep the back of the throat from collapsing are not very high. There are several types of positive airway pressure (PAP) devices to provide the air flow under pressure, including a single level of pressure, two levels of pressure, and new so-called 'smart' devices. In continuous positive airway pressure (CPAP), both the inhaled and exhaled pressures are the same. An alternative is to use bi-level positive airway pressure in which the inhaled and exhaled pressures can each be individually set. The PAP devices (sometimes called non-invasive ventilation devices) are set to deliver the level(s) of pressure found to be effective during an overnight sleep study. The 'smart' devices are capable of measuring the flow of air continuously and deliver an appropriate level of pressure to keep the airway open and which may vary from moment to moment during the night.

Supplemental oxygen is often used to treat falls in oxygen level during the night. If you use supplemental oxygen at night as part of your COPD treatment, and also have sleep apnea, your doctor needs to take special precautions. In some people, supplemental oxygen during sleep can actually reduce the drive to breathe, thereby creating hypopneas or apnea. Sometimes the supplemental oxygen might actually cause a reduction of oxygen and an increase in carbon dioxide in the blood. If these problems are found, your doctor may decide to use some form of non-invasive ventilation, such as bi-level positive airway pressure, when oxygen is administered.

Surgery is often considered as a treatment for apnea. Surgical removal of excess tissue from the back of the throat is rarely successful and carries only modest long-term results. The use of laser surgery has not proven successful for the treatment of apnea. The use of radio-frequency energy (Somnoplasty™) to modify tissues has not yet demonstrated success for treating apnea, although reports on experience with this method are expected to be published. Some people may receive full or partial relief when structures in the nose are corrected to eliminate restrictions of airflow, e.g., correcting a deviated septum. There are

Figure 31   CPAP and bi-level positive airway pressure devices

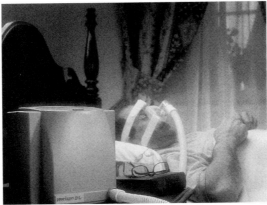

This DeVilbiss Horizon Bi-Level® Model 7355D is a bi-level positive airway device that is used to treat obstructive sleep apnea.

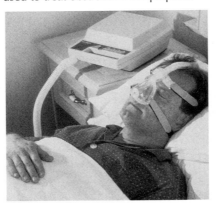

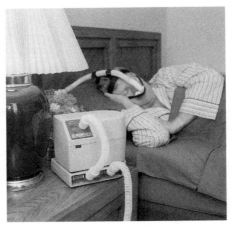

The Sullivan V Elite® CPAP system with Sullivan Mirage® Nasal Mask System is used to treat obstructive sleep apnea.

The Mallincrodt KnightStar™ 320 bi-level system is used to treat obstructive sleep apnea.

special considerations before surgery for people with COPD and people with sleep apnea should be sure that their surgeon and anesthesiologist are aware of the need to avoid collapse of the airway before or after surgery. See *Considerations Before Surgery* on page 197.

If losing weight and trying CPAP or bi-level airway pressure have been conclusively shown to be ineffective, there is a surgical solution called *tracheostomy.* It is a surgical opening in the trachea, through the neck. This opening in the neck bypasses the upper airway obstruction in the throat or back of the mouth. Supplemental oxygen can also be provided through a tracheostomy. A tracheostomy may be made at a location similar to that shown for *Transtracheal oxygen delivery* on page 100. However, the catheter or tube for the tracheostomy may be larger. The tracheostomy can be closed off during daily activities permitting normal speech and eating, although caution must be used to avoid letting in water (showering, water sports).

Sex and COPD

A sexual problem has been appropriately defined by Calderone as "the malfunction of any part of an individual's organism or life in such a way as to cause his sexual life to appear to him unrewarding or inadequate, or to be potentially harmful to another individual and therefore himself."

People with COPD, male and female, of differing ages, have relationships and sexual needs. These must be addressed in a total rehabilitation process. Sex usually means sexual intercourse. Sex means many things to different people. It can be purely biological, relating to physical pleasure, performance, and self, or it may be much broader, including the whole person, attitudes, gender differences, personality, and intimacy. People with COPD need to understand the issues related to sex and their chronic disease.

Sexual functions can be affected by chronic illness in a variety of ways, including impotence. Shortness of breath or dyspnea is the major complaint of people with COPD, limiting physical exertion and presenting a major obstacle to active sexual intercourse. Coping skills have a lot to do with successful sexual function and behavior as COPD advances. At present, sexual function with COPD cannot be predicted with pulmonary function studies.

The person with COPD confronts three distinct aspects of sexual functioning:

- *Impersonal skills:* limited exercise, chronic cough, sputum production and medication side effects
- *Intrapersonal skills:* decreased self-esteem, altered masculine/feminine roles and anxiety
- *Interpersonal obstacles between self and partner:* fear of sexual failure, embarrassment, or suppression of sexual desire.

However, many normal couples also face these obstacles, so this section doesn't cover all aspects of sexuality, but only some of the major issues facing people with COPD.

Explore your sexual knowledge and sexual attitudes. You and your partner may need to talk with each other, alone or in the company of a therapist or doctor. The attitude should be "sex-positive" for both of you. It is important that you both understand your physical limitations. Alternative, less physically-demanding positions for sex can be tried. Ask about them.

Some medications can cause sexual dysfunction. For example, some medicines for high blood pressure and other ailments can contribute to male impotence, including: diuretics, anticholinergics, antihistamines, antidepressives, sedatives and alcohol. Other medications known to decrease libido or the desire for sex are *antihypertensives* (high blood pressure medication).

Sexual impotence has also been linked to obstructive sleep apnea. Be aware of the possibility of drug-induced dysfunction and be ready to speak with your doctor if you have problems. There is at least one medication for male impotence, Viagra®. Ask your doctor.

Stress and depression are also linked with sexual dysfunction. These issues are not unique, many people with chronic diseases encounter them at various times.

Support groups such as Better Breathers Clubs and AWAKE discuss relevant issues and can provide guidance and referral. Your doctor may be an excellent resource. Pulmonary rehabilitation programs generally include information and counseling for sexual functioning.

Suggestions for Lovemaking

- Be physically and emotionally rested.
- Start slowly and take your time.
- Choose the best breathing time.
- Avoid alcohol and large meals before sex.
- Use medications and oxygen appropriately.
- Use positions which conserve energy.
- Be creative and romantic.

Even in today's enlightened environment, sex is a subject that is difficult to talk about. In my experience with COPD support groups, it is a topic that needs discussion, but even in the sharing atmosphere of a meeting, is mostly considered taboo. This may be because lung support groups include both sexes, include many single men and women of varied ages. As opinions, philosophy, and problems in sexual function are usually considered very personal, the embarrassment-factor is high. Help is available from the National Jewish Medical Research Center in a booklet in their Education series, "Being Close"[1]. It is a frank, well-presented little book on intimacy for COPD people to share with your partner. I highly recommend it to help you adjust to the changes that occur with chronic illness, and to provide you with information that will allow you to relax and cope with both emotional and physical restriction. Call NJMRC at 1- 800-222-LUNG to request a copy of "Being Close".

JVT

---

1. "Being Close" National Jewish Medical and Research Center. Denver

8 Exercise and Nutrition

Exercise

More Frequently-asked Questions

I have arthritis. Is there a program for me?

Yes. Talk with your doctor. If you start a program on your own, first decide which activities and which joints are more painful, or more likely to be injured. Take your medications before you exercise, consider using warm damp compresses on affected joints. Start slowly and build up gradually. If pain develops, stop exercising. If pain always develops with a particular exercise, change the exercise.

I have diabetes. Can I exercise?

Yes. Aerobic exercise helps control diabetes. First, you should be on a steady program of medical intervention, monitoring and diet. Then select a time of day to exercise. This is more important for diabetics than for others. Perform exercise according to your doctor's recommendations. This may include treadmill walking or exercise biking. Monitor your responses to exercise and be aware of changes. Some people may need extra sugar before or after exercise. A program of regular exercise and weight loss helps control diabetes and may make it possible for some to control diabetes without insulin.

I have had open heart surgery to bypass obstructed arteries. Will exercise help me?

Yes. An aerobic exercise conditioning program will help the recovery process, improve your physical abilities, reduce stress, and demonstrate that you can resume an active and productive life. Further, if you have high lipids (cholesterol), exercise helps to lower them. Check with your doctor before starting.

I have heart disease. Are there exercises to avoid?

> Avoid exercises where maximum effort is used, such as lifting heavy objects and straining. Aerobic training is preferred for people with heart, lung, and blood-vessel disease. Check with your doctor before starting.

I have difficulty taking my pulse. Is there another guide I could use for adjusting exercise intensity?

> If during the course of your activity you cannot hold a conversation with someone because of your breathing, you are probably working too hard. But this is not a replacement for determining your heart rate and maintaining your target heart rate levels.

I take breathing medications which affect my heart rate. Is there a way to monitor how hard I am working?

> If medications raise your heart rate, then when you begin to exercise the rate may significantly increase. In this case heart-rate monitoring still works. But if heart-rate monitoring doesn't work there are a couple of alternatives:
> - Slow down or rest. If you are working too hard you will not be able to hold a conversation.
> - Undergo a formal exercise test where exact work loads are measured and an exercise prescription is created for you based on work load (for example, speed and grade of walking).

Some of the new treadmills have exercise programs built in. What should I know about these programs?

> The manufacturer has installed various exercise programs to make it easier for a person in normal health to exercise and to add some variety to exercise. With COPD, these programs may be too strenuous. If you use a program, be sure that the highest work load programmed is not more than is recommended for you. Talk with your doctor.

Should I warm up and cool down?

> Yes. Stretching exercises performed as part of the warm up and cool down will increase joint flexibility and reduce the risk of joint and muscle injury.

Will exercise training harm my lungs?

> No. Data supports exercising for people with lung disease.

How can I increase the number of calories burned?

> Lengthen exercise time and frequency. Heavier people who walk or jog burn more calories than lighter people. See Table 13, "Calories burned per minute by a 150 pound person," on page 131, and Table 14, "Calories burned per hour by a 150 pound person," on page 132. These are estimates of calorie expenditure.

Myths About Exercise

Exercising makes you tired.

> Most people feel that as they condition their bodies they have more energy than before. The body becomes more efficient.

Exercising takes too much time.

Regular exercise takes only 30 to 50 minutes, three to five days a week. At first it seems hard to stay with a regular program. However, after a short time regular exercise becomes part of your regular routine.

All exercises give the same benefit.

Regular brisk exercise helps condition the heart, lungs and muscles. Examples are walking, cycling, jogging.

Muscle-strengthening exercises are good for aging people. As we age we lose muscle strength and our muscles become less efficient. Examples are weight training using light to moderate weight resistance, exercising with elastic bands which add resistance or other devices which allow for full range of motion at the joint, and resistance for working muscle groups.

For those with lung disease, training respiratory muscles for breathing may be important. This is commonly referred to as breathing retraining or resistive respiratory muscle training.

The older you are the less exercise you need.

With age we tend to become less active. Over time we lose strength and endurance due to inactivity or lack of quality activity. With chronic disease such as COPD, we tend to adopt a more sedentary life style at an earlier age to avoid shortness of breath. This accelerates the deconditioning process and makes even the simplest task hard. You still need to exercise. With a tailored program of activity you can regain your fitness even in the presence of such conditions as COPD.

You have to be an athlete to exercise.

Nothing is farther from the truth. We all need quality exercise no matter what our condition. Find an exercise program that conditions your body and at the same time is enjoyable. Everyone can and should exercise regularly. For people with COPD, a little more planning may be needed to balance medications with an exercise program.

I am sick and I should not exercise.

People with chronic disease such as COPD, heart disease or diabetes can and should exercise regularly. In a period of acute illness, exercise should be reduced or possibly avoided until the illness is resolved. Your doctor can tell you when to resume. When you do, start slowly and build back to where you were.

As a member of a lung support group, I've seen how important fitness and exercise programs are. I've witnessed many friends as they've moved from depressed, inactive states of sickness and resignation, through pulmonary rehabilitation, to more vital, active, and improved lives.

JVT

Deconditioning

Many people believe that because their lung disease cannot be reversed there is nothing they can do to improve their life. This is not the case. With any long term disease comes inactivity, which causes weakened muscles called *deconditioning*. Even the early astronauts, who were in superb physical shape, suffered from deconditioning after space flight without exercise. This problem was recognized and corrected in later flights with vigorous exercise programs. When someone with COPD has become deconditioned, or weak through lack of activity, that weakness can be corrected with increased activity.

How do you know that you are deconditioned? It may be suspected if your ability to perform normal activities is less than expected for your degree of lung disease. The chief symptom of both lung disease and deconditioning is shortness of breath. Deconditioning can be confirmed by testing you in an exercise laboratory to discover how much your lungs limit you and how much your muscles do. This testing will also show heart disease which may make it dangerous for you to exercise.

Reconditioning improves your ability to perform activities with less difficulty breathing. Exercise training will be difficult at times, and dyspnea unpleasant, but fortunately, benefits are usually obvious to you within the first one to two weeks of a good program and gradually increase.

Exercise for Health—Even With COPD

Health is the number one reason why so many people participate in regular exercise. Social and recreational reasons have lower priorities. Research has shown that regular, moderately vigorous exercise can improve the body's ability to use oxygen during exertion, can make the heart pump more efficiently, reduce blood pressure, and increase the amount of work you can do without being short of breath. Exercise also helps the body to burn calories and control body weight, stop smoking and control the weight gain which often follows.

COPD makes some simple activities difficult and difficult ones impossible. Therefore, there is confusion about the role and amount of exercise needed. We encourage exercise to combat the ill effects of COPD with an exercise program appropriate for you. In general, exercise is used as a treatment in lung disease to:

- Increase stamina
- Reduce or control shortness of breath
- Counter the effects of aging and deconditioning.

Exercise can significantly add to your quality of life. Pulmonary rehabilitation programs available in many hospitals and rehab facilities help to educate you about your lung disease, and to teach closely-supervised exercises. This helps you to regain as much physical conditioning and muscle toning as possible. Even if you can't get into a formal rehabilitation program, your doctor may be able to help you find a qualified person to develop a suitable set of exercises and activities that will help you improve your quality of life.

Medical Considerations for Exercise Participants

Exercise is recommended for a wide variety of medical conditions, it is safe and a necessary part of medical treatment for most people.

WARNING: **Get a medical release from your doctor before starting an exercise program.**

WARNING: **These guidelines are examples and may not be appropriate for you. Ask for exercise training guidelines from your own doctor.**

Your doctor may want you to take a stress test on a treadmill or bicycle before starting a program of regular exercise, to see what work load is appropriate, your physical ability at the time of testing, and any abnormal events during testing.

If you have been prescribed a medication for your heart or blood pressure, consult your doctor before exercising. There are medications which affect the heart's ability to speed up or slow down in certain circumstances, and some heart and blood-pressure medicines change heart rates. Other medications, such as theophylline or the bronchodilators, may increase heart rate. There may be others as well.

If you become ill, reduce or stop your training.

If you have been out for several training periods, when you resume reduce your training and build back up to where you left off. Be aware of what your body is telling you and use some common sense.

From my own experience with moderately-severe COPD, I've learned to expect a decrease in my general body conditioning after an exacerbation, or lung infection. Bouts of illness like this take a toll... with fever, increased shortness of breath and sputum production resulting in muscle weakness and loss of tone. Don't despair if you are faced with a setback in your exercise program. Just gradually work your way back to the previous state of conditioning and exercise tolerance. As soon as you are able to resume your exercise program (even on a limited basis), do so, in order to begin the process of building yourself back up. The more time you stay off your exercise regimen, the more loss you will notice in overall fitness, including your breathing. *JVT*

Limits on Exercise with COPD

The limiting factor for you in exercising with COPD is the ability to move air in and out of your lungs fast enough to meet increased demands. You may get an unbearable feeling of difficulty breathing, and stop the activity. This is a decision that your body makes for you, called *symptom-limited exercise.* As lung disease gets worse, less oxygen gets into your blood through your diseased lungs. This *hypoxemia* or lack of oxygen in your blood may be present only during extreme or heavy exertion at first, but with severe disease, hypoxemia may be present even when you're not exercising at all, even at rest.

The normal response is to limit or avoid activities which bring discomfort. Unfortunately, *deconditioning* through lack of activity only makes muscles weak from lack of use. The process of correcting this is *reconditioning* or *conditioning.*

Although basic principles of exercise conditioning are well developed and understood, there is controversy about the best training for people whose muscles are weak from lack of use. How much exercise is right? How hard do you push people to exercise, especially if there is lung disease? The approach presented here is based on many years of working with COPD people and attempts to match exercise with your needs and capabilities.

As a total training concept, we review basic bodily adjustments for exercise, the principles for every level, how to determine your resting and exercise heart rates, and how to use weight training. Exercise conditioning and training, and breathing retraining are all parts of a good exercise program.

There are many practical and medical issues related to exercise for people with pulmonary disease. These include: severity of the disease, need for supplemental oxygen, and any medical conditions that might limit exercise.

To determine which recommendations are most suited to your degree of COPD, you need to get your disease classification from your doctor: mild, moderate or severe. Classification reflects your difficulty in breathing and is measured by lung-function testing. See *Breathing Tests* on page 57.

Rules

General rules for exercising:

- When starting a program of regular physical activity don't overdo it.
- Be realistic with the goals you set for yourself.
- Start with an easy pace and gradually build up over weeks or months.
- Know your medical condition before starting an exercise program.
- Plan your medication and eating habits.
- Dress appropriately for the exercise.
- Wear good jogging shoes for walking or jogging.
- When stretching use smooth controlled movements.
- Start slowly and build up.
- If an exercise hurts, modify or don't perform it.
- Set up a regular exercise program and stay with it.
- Warm-up and cool down before and after each session.
- Use bronchodilators 30 minutes before exercise.
- Pay attention to what your body is telling you.
- Exercise at a capacity that will improve function yet will not place you at risk.
- Try to stay active throughout the rest of the day.
- Keep track of your progress.
- If your medical condition changes, check with your doctor.
- Do exercise with supplemental oxygen if it has been prescribed.

Exercise and Your Body

It is important for you to remain as active as possible. The two types of conditioning are:

- Aerobic or moderate-intensity, long-duration exercise
- Anaerobic or high-intensity, short-duration exercise.

Aerobic simply means that the exercise only goes on while the muscle is supplied with enough oxygen to serve as fuel. Examples of aerobic or rhythmic exercises are walking, jogging, swimming, cycling, or almost any activity which can be performed for a long period of time. *Anaerobic* exercise, on the other hand, requires the muscle to contract or work when there is a lack of oxygen. This occurs when you exert maximally for a short time or when a normal respiratory system cannot supply oxygen to working muscles. Examples are lifting heavy objects, strenuous weight lifting, sprinting, or pushing against an immovable object. Each form of training benefits muscles and organs.

Aerobic training conditions the heart, lungs and other organs for *endurance*. It strengthens skeletal muscles of arms and legs only if they are used in the exercise. The use of light weights with many contractions over a period of time is endurance or aerobic training. Aerobic exercise also burns calories and helps reduce shortness of breath.

Anaerobic training promotes skeletal muscle *strength* and adds size to the muscle. With maximal or near-maximal skeletal muscle contractions, blood pressure and heart rate may increase significantly. Avoid this if you have high blood pressure.

What Happens When You Exercise

When you participate in *any* activity your body senses change and prepares itself. The most notable changes are increases in heart rate and breathing. A higher heart rate means that more blood is pumped to the muscles, blood rich in foods and oxygen necessary for muscle contraction. Increased breathing increases exchange of oxygen and carbon dioxide, because of increased blood circulation to the lungs. This blood is moved by the beating action of the heart to the muscles where it will be used. Many other adjustments take place as well. Nervous system activity increases, hormones are released from various areas in the body, blood vessels change their size, some becoming smaller, some larger, and food stored in the body is released in preparation for activity. And this is only the beginning.

Heart rate

Heart rate or *pulse* is the number of beats your heart makes in one minute. Find your pulse at the wrist on the thumb side or in the neck below the jaw. Count the number of beats in one minute.

Figure 32   Taking your pulse

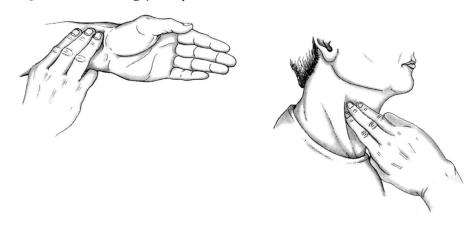

Find your pulse at the wrist on the thumb side or in the neck below the jaw.

A shorter method for estimating heart rate is the 10-second method. Locate and count your pulse for 10 seconds. Then multiply that number by 6 to get heart rate in beats per minute. For example, for 12 pulses in 10 seconds, heart rate is 72 bpm. If you begin to exercise, and your next pulse count is 25, your heart rate is 150 bpm.

Knowing how fast your heart is beating is also useful in discussing problems with your doctor or nurse. This information is most useful if you have an idea of your average heart rate from day to day. To help you calculate your heart rate use the heart-rate table. Count your pulse for ten seconds then look up your rate and corresponding heart rate (See *Calculate your heart rate*).

Table 11: Calculate your heart rate

Number of beats in 10 seconds	10	11	12	13	14	15	16	17	18	19
Your heart rate (beats per minute)	60	66	72	78	84	90	96	102	108	114
Number of beats in 10 seconds	20	21	22	23	24	25	26	27	28	29
Your heart rate (beats per minute)	120	126	132	138	144	150	156	162	168	174

Heart rate increases as work intensity increases with a peak value for each person. When you exercise, your heart rate (HR) increases to keep pace with your increased activity. The figure shows a typical heart rate response to increasing exertion on a motor-driven treadmill. As you walk faster and do more work, your heart rate increases, indicating how hard you are working. As you age, your heart's ability to pump strongly at high speed decreases. Maximum heart rate decreases with age. The older you are the lower your heart rate during strenuous activity. Some people may never achieve estimated maximal heart rate, while others may surpass estimated values.

Table 12: Maximum heart rate decreases with age

Age	40	45	50	55	60	65	70	75	80
Estimates of maximum heart rate (beats per minute)	180	175	170	165	160	155	150	145	140

These maximums (based on the formula 220 -age= bpm maximum) may typically vary by 10-15 bpm. and are representative of published studies, however your own rate can best be determined by your doctor and a treadmill test. Your heart rate maximum may be affected by your age, level of activity, and many other health factors.

Blood pressure

Blood pressure propels blood through the arteries, arterioles and capillaries, the blood vessels which lead away from the heart into the body. If you are nervous, upset or have been exercising, your systolic pressure may be elevated. This is a normal response. Figure 33 shows blood pressure response to increasing exercise stress or work load performed on a treadmill. If your blood pressure response is normal, the systolic pressure will increase as work load increases while the diastolic pressure doesn't change much. Persons with abnormal conditions, such as hypertensive (high) or hypotensive (low) will have quite different systolic pressures in response to exercise.

Breathing or Respiration

Respiration or breathing rate increases with exercise. Breathing rate is the number of breaths per minute. Depth of breathing is the amount of air moved in and out with each breath. Rate of breathing is usually not more than 60 breaths per minute even in the most vigorous adult exercise. For normal people, inability to increase breathing doesn't limit exercise capacity. Normally, exercise ability is limited by the heart's ability to keep up. However, with lung disease such as COPD, exercise capacity may be limited by breathing.

Figure 33   Systolic blood pressure responds to increasing workload

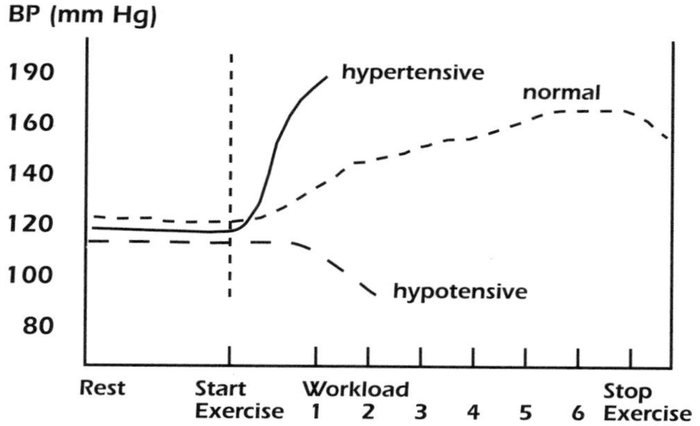

Systolic blood pressure: In a normal person, the value increases as the exercise workload increases, and declines when exercise stops.

Systolic blood pressure (hypertensive): Rapid, excessive rise in response to exercise.

Systolic blood pressure (hypotensive): A person with this condition can get dizzy or even pass out in response to exercise.

Body fat

Body fat is storage of calories eaten in excess of what you need. People with COPD may be overweight, of normal weight or underweight. For those of you who are underweight, exercise will stimulate your appetite. Just sitting around can lead to decreased appetite, less eating, and malnutrition. Eat frequently and try to eat high-calorie foods. Watch your body weight and percent of fat stores for improvements.

Excess body fat is associated with increased heart disease and may cause problems with breathing. Excess body fat places an extra burden on all of your systems, so that your body works harder to carry out each activity.

Body weight, body fat, and lean body weight are different measurements. If you weigh yourself daily, you know your weight, but not what percent of your weight is fat or how much lean body weight you have.

Lean body weight, on the other hand, is the amount of good active tissue in your body. This is the healthy side of what is measured on the bathroom scale. As a rule, young men and women should be less than 20% and 25% body fat, respectively. You can estimate your body fat through simple measurements. See *Body Fat Measurement* on page 221.

Examples

A 6'2" and 260 lb. male athlete weighs a lot and more than some of the height/weight published tables. Yet he has only 16% body fat. He may be overweight according to a table, but not obese.

A 5'2" 110 lb. female has 30% body fat. This female is small, and has excess body fat.

Exercising to Lose Weight

One pound of fat is approximately equal to 3500 stored calories. So to lose a pound of fat you must burn 3500 calories more than you normally eat. Fat reduction should be a gradual process not an overnight goal. Most diets or fast reducing plans simply remove water from the body to reduce weight and have nothing to do with reducing fat weight.

Body composition changes constantly. Consider a good example of how the body adjusts to changes in exercise habits.

Examples

A 60 year old male buys a treadmill and starts a conditioning program with the advice of his doctor. At the start, his body weight is 220 lb., height 5'11", body fat 27%. He is starting the conditioning program to reduce body fat and control weight. After two weeks of training he weighs himself and finds that his weight is now 227 pounds, an increase of seven pounds. What is going on?

He decides to measure his percent body fat again and notes that it is now 25% compared to 27% two weeks before, a loss of 2% body fat. He has also reduced his waistline by three inches.

What happened was that through training, this once-sedentary male increased his lean body weight or muscle weight, and decreased his fat weight. Because muscle weighs more than fat, the bathroom scale simply reported all it could, a weight gain.

Six months later his body weight is 200 pounds, his percent body fat is 15%, and his waistline reduced by a total of 6.5 inches.

This is a good example of how the body adjusts to changes in exercise habits.

Calories and Exercise

Energy is the basis of life, provided by the food we eat and measured in *calories*. Each of us has a base metabolic rate which is the minimum number of calories we need to eat in order to live. Add calories for activities, such as sitting, reading, walking, typing, homemaking, driving, and exercise. The harder you work, the more calories you need. If you eat more calories than you use on a daily basis, you become heavier because you store the calories as fat in various areas of your body: different areas for men and for women.

One reason for starting an exercise program is to regain control over body composition, the amount of fat related to the amount of muscle. The following table is a guide for burning the calories that healthy people don't need. If you have moderate to severe COPD, the values in the table are too low. This is because you have to work harder to breathe when you have lung disease, and burn more calories than a healthy person. Also, calories continue to be burned after the exercise session. So if you burn an extra 300 calories per day, and don't increase the number of calories you eat, you can lose a pound of fat in less than two weeks. Weight lost in this way usually stays off.

Calorie Expenditure Estimates

Table 13: Calories burned per minute by a 150 pound person

Activity	Calories/minute
Aerobics	6.6
Bicycling	6.35
Running	13.2
Swimming	8.1
Walking	3.8

Exercising to Add Weight

For those who wish to add weight, a combination of exercise and added calories provides the greatest benefit. This is because the weight that is added is mostly muscle and good functional tissue, not fat. One strategy is to increase the number of meals you eat in a day. Another is to eat frequent snacks. Combined with a good exercise program, the additional calories replenish burned calories, and build muscle tissue. A snack following exercise is also good, as this adds calories, and converts sugars to useable complex sugar or *glycogen*, that is stored and used by muscles.

Exercise and Conditioning Concepts

There are four ingredients in a successful training or conditioning program:

- *Intensity* or how hard you exercise
- *Duration* or how long you exercise at a single time
- *Frequency* or how many times per week you exercise
- *Mode* or which exercise(s) you do.

Each is important and each varies depending on the goal of the conditioning program. Since you are concerned with cardiopulmonary health, the focus of this section is in this area. If you have advanced or severe COPD, your exercise program will most likely be limited by shortness of breath. Ask your doctor about exercise guidelines based on your medical history, laboratory tests and specific needs. Exercise is not easy, often boring, and your muscles may ache the day after, until you become accustomed to the program. This takes from one to two weeks if you are faithful. Don't get discouraged. The aches and pains will most likely go away.

Intensity

Intensity is measured by heart rate during exercise.

Subtract your age from 220 (220 - age = maximum predicted heart rate).

Then multiply by a percent between 70% and 85%, depending on how active you are and whether or not you have heart problems (maximum heart rate x% = target heart rate).

Table 14: Calories burned per hour by a 150 pound person

Activity	Calories/hr.	Activity	Calories/hr.
Archery	264	Golf (without a cart)	348
Badminton	396	Gymnastics	270
Basketball	564	Judo	798
Billiards	174	Running 11.5 min.per mile 9 min. per mile 8 min. per mile 7 min. per mile 6 min. per mile 5.5 min. per mile	552 786 852 936 1038 1182
Canoeing "leisure"	180	Skiing, cross country hard snow Level, moderate speed Level, walking Uphill, maximum speed	486 582 1116
Card playing	102	Skiing, downhill soft snow Leisure (F) Leisure (M)	402 450
Carpentry, general	210	Snowshoeing, soft snow	678
Circuit-training	756	Squash	864
Climbing hills w/no load w/5 kg. load w/10 kg. load	492 528 570	Table tennis	276
Dancing Ballroom "Twist" "Wiggle"	210 420	Tennis	444
Fishing	252	Volleyball	204
Football	540		
Ax chopping, fast	1212		
Ax chopping, slow	348		
Gardening Digging Hedging Mowing Raking	516 312 456 222		

Example for a 60-year-old:

His estimated maximum heart rate is 160 beats per minute (220 - 60 = 160 BPM).

His estimated training heart rate is between 112 and 136 beats per minute (BPM) depending on regularity of exercise.

Rarely exercises 220 - 60 = 160 BPM x 70% = 112 BPM training target (lower limit).

Regularly exercises 220 - 60 = 160 BPM x 85% = 136 BPM training target (upper limit).

Figure 34   Zones of training or training avoidance

Not exercising to a good level	Target exercise zone	Over the target limit	Theoretical area
Resting heart rate			
80 bpm	70% 112 bpm	85% 136 bpm	160 bpm	220 bpm

Duration

Duration is usually 20 to 45 minutes a day. With COPD, an even lower number may be appropriate to start.

Frequency

Frequency is usually at least three times a week. It is helpful to exercise daily, though you may have to slow down if you get too much muscle or joint soreness.

We discourage fewer days per week for two reasons:

• You are more prone to skeletal muscle soreness and injury.
• Good training habits are not developed so you don't get optimal benefit.

For more than three days per week, alternate easy and hard days of training. Also, vary the muscle group trained. For example, train on a treadmill three days and do upper-body exercise for another three days. Take a day off.

Mode

Mode of training is the type of exercises which you do. For many people with COPD, riding a stationary bicycle is easier than walking on a treadmill. Neither one of these will improve arm muscle endurance, and that is a problem in people with COPD. Additional exercises for the arms may be helpful.

Cardiovascular conditioning takes place when large muscle groups, like the legs, are exercised. However, you may have other areas of the body which should be trained, such as your upper body by swinging light weights while walking or jogging. As training is specific to the muscle groups performing the activity, if you lack strength or endurance in a particular muscle group, that's the group to train.

Start with treadmill walking.

Rules

• Set up a regular exercise program and stay with it.

- Set realistic goals.
- Use bronchodilators 30 minutes before exercise.
- Pay attention to what your body is telling you.
- Start each training session with a warm-up period of at least five minutes. Activities during this period should be focused at gradually increasing heart rate from resting levels to low training threshold and increasing joint flexibility. Start out slowly and increase gradually.
- Stretch both large and small muscle groups.
- Never use a bouncing motion while stretching.
- Start slowly and build up.
- Exercise to improve function, but not to take risks.
- If you notice pain, slow down. If you have severe pain, stop. Get professional help if necessary.
- End each training session with a five-minute cool down.
- Try to stay active during the rest of the day.
- Keep track of your progress.
- Choose exercise activities that you enjoy.

A typical training session (*Typical aerobic training session* on page 134) includes a warm-up, a period of aerobic activity at the training zone, and a cool down.

Figure 35   Typical aerobic training session

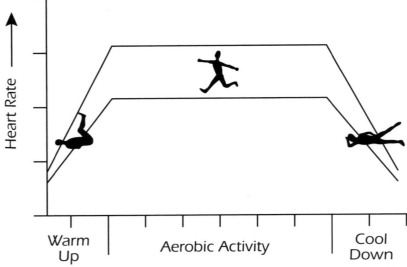

A typical training session includes a warm-up, a period of aerobic activity at the training zone and a cool down.

Dress for Exercise

Appropriate dress is important for exercise. Use a good pair of running shoes for walking, jogging or running. As running shoes are some of the best engineered shoes on the market today, spend a reasonable amount of money for them. The cost will be well worth it to avoid problems with your feet, ankles, knees, hips, or back related to improper shoes.

Figure 36   Selecting a shoe

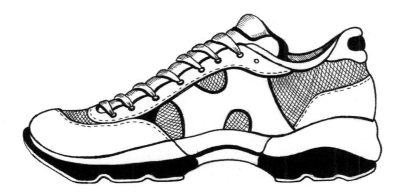

Appropriate dress is important for exercise. Use a good pair of running shoes for walking, jogging or running.

Before buying, we recommend that you read *Consumer Reports* or *Runners World* magazine for their yearly shoe ratings. After selecting several highly ranked shoes, try some on and select the one with the best fit. Wear these shoes only during exercise and not for daily activities. If you wear these shoes for daily activity, the support structure will lose its ability to absorb foot strikes and defeat the purpose of the shoe.

Wear loose-fitting clothing that is suitable for your climate, or for the environment where you exercise. Wear natural fabrics, such as 100% cotton, that breathe and allow good air circulation. In winter add layers of clothing. In summer take layers off. In the summer in hot climates, it is best to exercise in the early morning when the heat is low. In cooler months it is best to exercise in the evening, when it is warmer.

If you exercise indoors, dress in comfortable, loose-fitting clothing. For treadmill or cycle exercise, you may need a fan in the room to circulate air and help your body to cool through evaporation of perspiration.

Never wear clothing which blocks the body's ability to cool itself. This simply increases water loss and may give you heat exhaustion, heat stroke or other medical problems. Contrary to belief, suits which trap heat do not help to lose body fat. They simply decrease body weight through loss of water, which is quickly restored by drinking fluids or eating.

Cool dry air can cause some people to wheeze. If you have to exercise in cool dry air and you wheeze, wear a face mask. A face mask traps warm moist air as you breath out. When you breath in, cool air is warmed and moisture added from the moisture trapped in the face mask.

Aerobic Training

As you train aerobically, your body becomes better conditioned, improving the efficiency with which it works. One proof is gradual reduction of your heart rate. For example, to walk at two miles per hour on the treadmill might have given you a heart rate of 120 bpm before you started training. After training for a while, walking at that same speed might only require a heart rate of 110 bpm because you are in better condition. As your heart and blood vessels become stronger, they become more efficient so that your heart pumps more blood with each beat, having to make fewer beats to provide the same supply.

As your heart and blood vessels become more efficient, gradually increase the work load at which you train, to maintain training intensity. The increase in work load will vary depending upon your training response. For advanced COPD, there will be a ceiling reached when you are unable to increase breathing any further. As your body conditions itself, your heart and muscles become more efficient in using the limited resources available. You can increase your workload gradually, relying on changes in breathing, rather than heart rate as a guide to how much you can exercise. Some breathing medications increase heart rate so that heart rate is not a good guide for exercise intensity. If you have questions, ask your doctor.

Breathing techniques during exercise

Use two breathing techniques for shortness of breath while exercising: pursed-lips breathing and diaphragmatic breathing. See *Tools for Better Breathing* on page 45.

Weight Training

Recent data suggest that strength training can help to reverse chronic weakness. Regular aerobic training with a weight-training program may improve muscle strength and endurance.

For the greatest gains in *strength*, lift an object weighing almost as much as the maximum amount you can lift with the muscles you wish to strengthen. *Endurance strength* training uses weights equal to 50% to 70% of your best lift weight. Perform eight to twelve repetitions with this amount of weight, probably doing three or more cycles, then resting before the next three. Maintain as near normal breathing as possible and don't hold your breath while lifting.

Weight training is very important if you have moderate to severe COPD and shortness of breath associated with arm activity.

- Use very light weights to improve the strength and endurance of arm and shoulder muscles: one to three pound weights to start.
- Start with as many repetitions as you are able, up to 15.
- Then, strive to complete three sets of 15 repetitions with appropriate rest intervals.
- As you may not be able to do this much to start with, start slowly and build up.
- When you are able to complete three sets of 15 repetitions for each arm, consider increasing the weight, by half-pound increments.
- Improvise weight training at little or no cost with one-pound objects around your house, such as old flour sacks filled with sand, or cans of food.

Training Results

As your condition improves, changes may include some or all of the following:

- Heart rate reduced at rest and during work. Heart is more efficient.
- Slower and deeper breathing. Breathing is more efficient.
- Shortness of breath reduced.
- Breathing easier.

- Mucus cleared during exercise.
- Reduced systolic blood pressure.
- Increased endurance.
- Less or improved body fat and greater lean body mass.
- Repositioning of body fat compartments (slimmer waist line).
- Increased sense of well being.
- Reduced stress and depression.
- Increased vigor.
- Better control of diabetes and hypertension.
- Decreased levels of triglycerides and total cholesterol.
- Increased HDL (good) cholesterol.

Many other changes may also occur as a result of aerobic conditioning.

Exercise Programs

Stretching Exercises

Stretching exercises can be used in the warm-up and cool-down periods (See page 138).

Exercise Program for Mild to Moderate COPD

As an example, you are a 40-year-old with mild to moderate COPD, not taking medications that prevent heart rate from increasing in exercise, and with no known heart disease. Your doctor agrees you should begin an exercise program using treadmill walking in the comfort of your home and suggests your program also include strength and flexibility training. Work with your doctor to set up a realistic entry level program that can build gradually based on ability to exercise. Your purpose is to be more active with less shortness of breath. You also wish to control your body weight and improve aerobic fitness. Your exercise plan initially would appear as follows.

WARNING: **This is an example program only. Check with your doctor for your own needs.**

Intensity with Mild to Moderate COPD

Keep the intensity level at about 70% for at least two weeks, until you achieve 40 minutes of continuous exercise. This allows your body time to become accustomed to the new exercise program and hopefully, prevent muscle soreness. Increase intensity by 10 bpm to a maximum of 153 BPM thereafter.

Your estimated maximum heart rate is 180 bpm (220 - 40 = 180 bpm).

Your estimated training heart rate is between 126 and 153 bpm depending on regularity of exercise.

Rarely exercises 220 - 40 = 180 bpm x 70% = 126 bpm training target (lower limit).

Regularly exercises 220 - 40 = 180 bpm x 85% = 153 bpm training target (upper limit).

Figure 37   Stretching exercises for warm-up and cool-down

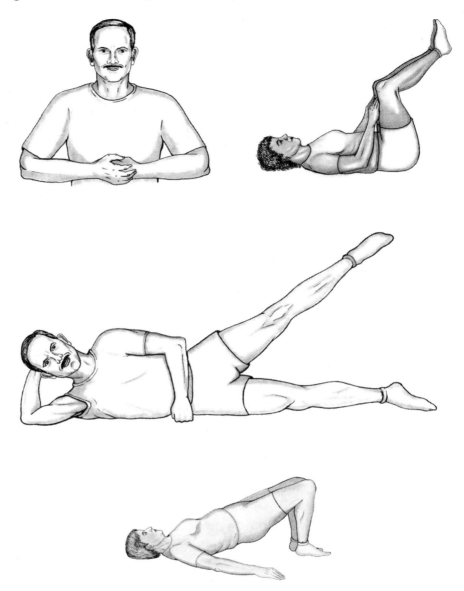

Stretching exercises can be used in the warm-up and cool-down periods.

Duration with Mild to Moderate COPD

At first you may find it difficult to complete 20 minutes of continuous exercise. Try two 10-minute periods with a rest period between. Your goal is 20 minutes of continuous exercise. After a week or two, try to increase duration in 2-minute increments. then increase by five minutes every two weeks to a maximum of 40 minutes of continuous exercise.

As a rule, you should try for 40 to 45 minutes of exercise before you increase intensity.

Frequency with Mild to Moderate COPD

Train at least three days per week on alternating days. This will encourage good conditioning.

Increase to four times per week as intensity and duration increase.

Exercise Program for Moderate to Severe COPD

If you have moderate to severe COPD, you know that you cannot exercise without difficulty. You cannot get enough air in and out of your lungs as fast as you need. You may also have oxygen shortage, stressing your heart and muscles. Because you are short of breath, you may have gradually cut down your activity level, which leads to muscle weakness.

As an example, you are a 65 year old man, diagnosed with COPD several years ago. You can't work around the house without getting very short of breath. Your doctor tells you it is severe. But so far, your doctor has not recommended that you get oxygen at home.

You take some breathing medications, including theophylline pills and two different inhalers, ipratropium and albuterol. You used to smoke heavily, over two packs a day, but quit when your lung disease was diagnosed five years ago. Because of your severe breathing problems, and because you are at high risk for heart disease due to your age and smoking history, your doctor is reluctant to allow you to exercise without being sure it is safe.

Your doctor did an exercise test recently and this test showed that your oxygen level did not get too low with the little bit of exercise that you were able to do. The test included electrocardiogram (ECG), blood pressure, and oxygen monitoring while walking on a treadmill or riding a stationary bicycle. This was the minimal evaluation to show the safety of exercise for you based on your heart, lung and muscle responses. Since using your arms is more difficult than using your legs, you were evaluated for arm work to see if it caused shortness of breath.

You remember to use your medications ahead of time, carry your inhaler for shortness of breath, and plan the exercise period.

WARNING: **This is an example program only. Check with your doctor for your own needs.**

Intensity for Moderate to Severe COPD

The intensity of exercise to start is established from the exercise test. Although the heart rate is usually used as the indicator for how much work you are doing, you had a different heart rate than expected during your exercise test. This sometimes happens because of your medicines, or because you get short of breath before you reach the heart rate you're aiming for.

Your goal is the heart rate the exercise prescription calls for: a certain speed and grade on the treadmill, a specific workload setting on a bicycle, and a set pace for walking out of doors or in a mall.

Your heart rate calculation is: 220 - 65 years = 155; 155 X 70% = 108 to start. Your target is 155 X 85% = 131 beats per minute (bpm).

You start exercise at about 108 bpm till you achieve 40 minutes of continuous exercise.

You increase intensity by 10 bpm to a maximum of 131 bpm thereafter.

When your respiratory medications elevate your heart rate before exercise, so that your resting heart rate is higher than your target heart rate, you can begin exercise, but raise your rate by ten BPM above your resting level.

Duration for Moderate to Severe COPD

Your starting target is 10 minutes per day for two weeks. You increase by five minutes every two weeks after that to a maximum of 40 minutes of continuous exercise. You intend to use two to three minutes of continuous exercise, then rest, continuing until you have accomplished the full duration.

Although your target duration at first is about 10 minutes, this is not possible for you in the first days, so you substitute four periods of five minutes at the prescribed intensity, with a rest period between each bout. When this is too difficult, you try two-minute exercise periods.

After several weeks, you are able to increase the duration by two-minute increments, increasing the length of time before you increase your intensity.

If you have great difficulty with this, don't feel bad. You are receiving a lot of benefit from what you are doing, but may have reached a limit to what your lungs can manage and be too short of breath to continue. This is the point where you can no longer increase your breathing to supply the oxygen for exercise, so you try to gradually increase your time at this level of exertion, using the breathing techniques in *Tools for Better Breathing* on page 45.

Frequency for Moderate to Severe COPD

You start with three times per week on alternating days, increasing to four times per week when intensity and duration requirements are satisfied.

Mode for Moderate to Severe COPD

As it is wise to alternate training different muscle groups, you train on a stationary bicycle without arm movements two days per week, and do treadmill walking the other two days.

You are short of breath when you try to carry groceries or packages, when you sweep or vacuum, or do some other activity involving your arms and upper body, so upper body conditioning can be of great benefit to you.

One training approach is to use light hand weights with good arm movement while walking, or a bicycle which has associated arm movements.

If you had other problems during the test, such as difficulty walking due to arthritis, or difficulty cycling because of back problems, your doctor may have recommended an adjusted mode or intensity based on your functional limitations. You may need other medications to permit you to exercise.

Nutrition

As COPD causes you to do more work to breathe than a normal person, even if you don't exercise, you must eat more to maintain your weight. At the same time, your desire and ability to eat without being uncomfortable may be reduced. For most people with COPD, the most important nutritional problem is not eating enough of the right kind of foods. In fact, weight loss is a major problem, difficult to correct.

With COPD, you need to eat between one and a half and two times as much as normal, but eat the right things and in the right way.

Eating

Eat lots of small meals instead of a few large ones. This prevents your abdomen getting tight and cutting off your breathing.

The choice of eating before or after exercise varies from person to person. Some people get an upset stomach or have shortness of breath when they eat before an exercise routine. Some feel listless and drained if they don't eat before exercise, whether a structured routine or activities such as gardening, lawn care, house work, or shopping.

Regardless of when you eat one thing is certain: the muscles of activity and breathing need feeding. Rules for eating are not hard and fast. Old myths such as "Don't exercise right after eating" have faded as evidence mounts that moderate exercise after eating has several advantages. Exercise may reduce the craving for food and this may help reduce caloric intake.

When to Eat

Exercising after meals is of particular value for some people. As research shows, exercise following a meal can burn more calories than exercise before a meal, by 15 to 30%. Exercise raises the body's metabolic rate and causes the body to continue to burn calories even after exercise. Most of the increase in calorie use occurs within the first hour after exercise, to restore the nutrients burned during exercise. This 'afterburn' may help reduce body fat in overweight people.

For other people, eating after exercise has some advantages. Eating following exercise has also been shown to replace glycogen, a stored sugar in muscle needed for quick energy for muscle contraction. In fact, for some it may be advisable to eat a candy bar after exercise so that the sugars can be converted to glycogen in the muscle.

With COPD, exercise before eating may cause less shortness of breath for two reasons:

- Less discomfort because the stomach is not loaded with food.
- Digestion requires an increase in the rate and depth of breathing which puts an increased strain on a person already having trouble with breathing during exercise.

Eating and Medical Conditions

Medical conditions may dictate when you can or must eat.

For example, diabetics need to exercise one to two hours after meals when blood sugars are high. People with diabetes who exercise early in the morning or three to four hours after a meal may use too much energy, resulting in low blood sugar. Diabetics should check blood glucose levels and adjust eating and exercise habits accordingly.

People with heart disease should do vigorous exercise before eating, but moderate exercise after eating, since blood tends to clot following eating. A brisk walk is better than assuming the couch potato position.

Reasons for Weight Loss and Not Eating

- With COPD, you use more energy than normal, almost like an athlete. You work every minute because of your lung problems. This particularly stresses the diaphragm. It can be weakened further if enough nutrition doesn't get to it to supply the extra demand. The diaphragm and all other muscles are damaged by weight loss and become even weaker.
- Problems with your breathing may lead to lack of appetite. If you are short of breath, eating may be too much work. Or it may just be too much work to prepare a meal, particularly if you live alone. You may notice more difficulty breathing after eating, when your stomach is fuller. Because of the loss of elastic tissue in the lungs, your lungs are overstretched and extend down into your stomach. When your stomach is full of food and especially if you have gas, your breathing is less comfortable.
- Depression, which is often present in people with COPD, decreases appetite. Nothing looks good and you don't want to eat. Loss of a loved one late in life may further decrease not only the desire for food, but also the desire to keep living.
- Poverty or a poor financial position may also cause problems. For many people on a fixed income, healthy food is neglected in order to pay for housing, buy medicines and get to the doctor's office.
- Some medications used to treat COPD may cause problems. Steroids such as prednisone or celestone, taken by mouth or injection, may cause diabetes. Even without diabetes, steroids may cause muscle damage and further weakness. This type of muscle damage may also happen while you are gaining weight, since steroids can cause excess fat.
- Poor teeth are a big factor in poor eating. This is more common in former or current smokers. Sometimes the teeth are still there, but broken and with cavities. Sometimes the teeth have been replaced by ill-fitting dentures. Poor teeth seem to decrease amount and quality of eating. For example, fresh fruit and vegetables are often impossible to eat without functional teeth.
- Arthritis can decrease your ability to move around and prepare meals.
- You may not like a prescribed diet, particularly if you have spent your life eating certain foods, prepared in certain ways. When you are told to cut down on salt or sugar or cornbread, food is just not the same. Fried and baked chicken are very different. For dessert fruit in its own juice may not be as appealing as coconut cream pie. Knowing that baked chicken is healthier doesn't make it taste better, so it is important to fit diet changes with your tastes, if at all possible. Now there are many more healthy choices in prepared foods than there used to be, and many recipes have been adapted for healthier eating, but still taste good.
- If any of these apply to you, discuss solutions with your doctor.

Determining Your Nutritional Health

Read the statements below. For yourself, or for someone you know, circle numbers in the YES column. Add the circled numbers to get the total nutritional score.

Table 15: Nutrition checklist[a]

	Yes
I have an illness or condition that made me change the kind and/or the amount of food I eat.	2
I eat fewer than two meals per day.	3
I eat few fruits, vegetables, or milk products.	2
I have three or more drinks of beer, liquor or wine almost every day.	2
I have tooth and mouth problems that make it hard for me to eat.	2
I don't always have enough money to buy the food I need.	4
I eat alone most of the time.	1
I take three or more different prescribed or over-the-counter drugs per day.	1
Without wanting to, I have lost or gained 10 pounds in the last 6 months.	2
I am not always physically able to shop for, cook for, and/or feed myself.	2
Total nutritional score	

a. Reprinted with permission from the Nutrition Screening Initiative. See *Copyrights and Trademarks* on page 244

If your total nutrition score is:

- 0-2 Good. Recheck your nutritional score in 6 months.
- 3-5 You are at moderate nutritional risk. See what can be done to improve your eating habits and lifestyle. Your office on aging, senior nutrition program, senior citizen's center, or health department can help. Recheck your score in three months.
- 6-21 You are at high risk. Bring this checklist the next time you see your doctor, dietician, or other qualified health care provider or social service professional. Talk with him/her about any problems you may have. Ask for help to improve your nutritional health.

Selecting Foods

Adequate nutrition or the ability to take in enough and the right kind of solid and liquid food to meet your body's needs, plays a crucial role in treating COPD. Selecting the right foods in the right amounts is critically important, as your lungs and the muscles that work them need more than the normal amount of energy. We are only beginning to understand some of the interactions between good nutritional practices and lung disease, but we do know that weight is a common problem in COPD. With weight loss comes muscle loss. If you are losing weight, you may need more calories. Even if you are at proper weight for your age and body, you may not be well nourished. If you are overweight, you may need to reduce calories.

Nutrients, or What is In Food

Nutrients are what all your cells, tissues, and organs need to reproduce, maintain and repair themselves. You must have nutrients to survive. The major groups of nutrients are: proteins, fats and carbohydrates (starches and sugars) and water. Other nutrients are tiny amounts of minerals and vitamins. All nutrients are needed by the body on a regular basis and in the proper amounts, to be digested and absorbed through the intestinal walls then carried in the blood to every part of your body. Many cells maintain a defense system called the *immune system*, that defends you against infection and which depend on good nutrition.

Food vs. supplements

No single food can supply all the nutrients you need. Eating a variety of foods provides a balance of protein, fats and carbohydrates with vitamins, minerals and fluids. Foods rich in nutrients are better for you than supplements, because critical trace elements may be missing in supplements, and many supplements do not provide nutritional elements in forms your body can use. Supplements are more expensive than a well-rounded diet, but proper use of supplements can be extremely helpful in some cases. Check with your doctor.

Calories

Calorie is the term used for the energy units supplied by food in proteins, fats and carbohydrates. During illness, your energy requirements increase. Therefore, what you eat today may have a significant effect on the way your body responds to illness and the speed at which you can return to good health.

Protein

Protein provides *amino acids* which build and repair tissues (especially muscle), create antibodies to fight infection, and assist in other functions. In a balanced diet that meets your energy demands, one-half gram of protein per pound of body weight is enough for an average adult. For example, if you weigh 100 pounds, you should eat 50 grams of protein daily. However, with lung disease, your protein requirements are higher.

Animal protein contains fat and cholesterol, while beans, grains and cereals contain little or none.

Fish, poultry, milk, dried peas and beans are all good sources of protein. Meat, eggs, nuts, and cheese are also good sources, but contain more fats.

Fats

Fat supplies calories for warmth and work. Fat also provides *essential fatty acids*, which are needed for growth, for hormone production (estrogen, testosterone, and others), for making the membrane around each cell in the body, and for storing vitamins which do not dissolve in water (A, D, E, K).

Your body stores extra calories as fat for a reserve energy source, to be used when you eat less than you need in a day. For many people, fat accumulates because they don't miss meals and always take in more nutrients than needed. For people with COPD, fat limitation may be less necessary than for healthy people.

Main food sources of fat are: butter, margarine, vegetable oil, shortening, salad dressing, fatty meats, nuts, whole-milk products such as cream and cheese.

- *Essential fatty acids*, Vitamins A, D, E, K. These are in foods such as fish liver and vegetable oils, fish, meat, eggs, whole milk products.
- *Fat soluble vitamins*. B Vitamins in foods such as nuts, eggs, meat, poultry and fish. Vitamin C in foods such as citrus fruits and dark-green-leafy vegetables.
- *Concentrated calories* in foods such as meat, fish, poultry, nuts, cheese, cream soups, milkshakes, chocolate, cakes, cookies, puddings.

Carbohydrates

Carbohydrates supply energy for heat and mechanical work such as lifting arms and legs, and walking. Carbohydrates are a relatively inexpensive and readily available source of calories. Some foods high in carbohydrates also provide vitamins, minerals, and fiber.

Diets high in carbohydrates give off carbon dioxide as a by-product, a drawback for people with COPD as extra carbon dioxide can increase shortness of breath by making you breathe deeper and faster.

Foods high in carbohydrates are: fruits, vegetables, flours, grains, breads, cereals, and pasta. Concentrated carbohydrates such as honey, molasses, syrups, and sugar do not have other essential nutrients, and can add a lot of calories without much bulk.

Vitamins and minerals

Vitamins and minerals start up, and control the activities of your cells, your *metabolism*, providing fine tuning and regulation of many cell activities. They do not provide calories or protein, and cannot replace food. The correct amount of many vitamins and minerals is supplied by a reasonable diet. Extra amounts are excreted as waste. However, some vitamins protect you against specific problems and extra amounts may be helpful. One good general multi-vitamin daily is now recommended for most people.

Anytime you are not eating much or you are not eating the correct combination of foods, you may not be taking in enough vitamins and minerals for your body's needs. Demand for vitamins and minerals increases during acute bouts of infection and as part of the chronic disease process when supplements may be helpful and you may benefit from a better diet plan which you can follow regularly.

If you are concerned that you are not getting adequate amounts of vitamins and minerals, talk with your doctor, and ask for referral to a good nutritionist.

Fiber

Fiber is essential to prevent constipation. It may also reduce the risk of cancer of the colon and may lower cholesterol. A good diet usually provides the fiber you need.

Be cautious about increasing fiber intake as it may increase the amount of gas produced by your intestine and worsen your shortness of breath.

Good sources of fiber are: raw fruits, vegetables, popcorn, nuts, bran, whole grain cereals and whole grain breads.

Liquids

Drink plenty of liquids every day, particularly water. This also helps prevent constipation.

Note on Laxatives

Because of poor nutrition and reduced exercise levels, constipation is a common complaint. Many Americans rely on laxatives over the years, but continual use of laxatives can prevent absorption of some nutrients and may require aggressive dietary intervention and retraining of normal bowel habits. If you use laxatives, talk with your doctor, or with a specialist in digestive disorders.

Nutritional Labeling

Recently, the food producers of America changed the labeling of food, to make comparison of products easier, and to give clearer nutritional information. The following example of the new nutritional label is from a box of vegetable crackers and is explained in *Label explanations* on page 147.

Table 16: Nutrition label sample

Serving size 11 crackers (30 G)
Servings per container about 5
Calories 140 calories from fat 50

Total fat	6 g	9%
Saturated fat	0.5 g	3%
Cholesterol	0 mg.	0%
Sodium	230 mg.	10%
Total Carbohydrate	19 G	6%
Dietary Fiber	1 g	4%
Sugars	1 g	
Protein	3g	
Vitamin A		2%
Vitamin C		0%
Calcium		0%
Iron		6%

Percent Daily Values are based on a 2,000 calorie diet. Your daily values may be higher or lower depending on your calorie needs

Calories	2,000	2,500
Total Fat	less than 85 G	80 g
Sat fat	less than 20 g	25 g
Cholesterol	less than 300 mg.	300 mg.
Sodium	less than 2,400 mg.	2,400 mg.
Total carbohydrate	300 g	375 g
Dietary fiber	25 g	30 g

How Much Fat?

Americans eat many fast foods rich in fats and calories and low in other nutrients. Most Americans can afford to lose some fat weight while maintaining or increasing muscle weight. Adding weight should be adding muscle, not fat, because muscle mass allows you to perform activities. Bigger muscles usually mean that tasks are easier. For example, with muscles in poor condition, a task is harder to complete and creates more shortness of breath than with improved muscle mass and strength.

Extra fat is like hauling around five, ten, fifteen or twenty pounds of baggage. A simple method, fairly accurate is given below for estimating how much you should weigh given your age, height, and sex. These values may vary as much as 10% above or below the values given.

Table 17: Label explanations

Serving size	Is your serving size the same as that listed? If you eat double the serving size you need to double the nutrient and caloric values. If you eat less, then reduce the values.
Calories	Are you overweight or underweight? Adjust calories to meet your needs.
Total carbohydrate	When you reduce your fat intake you can generally increase the calories from carbohydrates such as bread and potatoes. Choose solid foods over beverages, as solid foods contain important nutrients that may be missing in liquids.
Dietary fiber	Increase the amount of dietary fiber, if possible, but do it gradually, to prevent gas.
Protein	Most of us get enough protein.
Vitamins and minerals	Vitamins and minerals are best taken in as part of a good meal plan.
Total Fat	For many, fat intake should be limited. However, if you are losing weight with COPD, add some fat calories. Easing restrictions on fat may help increase your desire to eat by increasing the variety of foods available.
Saturated fat	Try to avoid saturated fat since these fats are closely linked to high cholesterol and heart disease.
Cholesterol	Limit cholesterol intake when possible. There are two sources of cholesterol. One source is in foods containing cholesterol, the other source is when the body makes cholesterol from saturated fats.
Salt	Salt contains sodium which can lead to ankle swelling and fluid retention. It may also cause high blood pressure. Limit the salt you add to foods, to less than 3,000 mg. per day. Fresh fruits and vegetables have almost no salt.
Daily value	Daily values are listed for people who eat 2,000 or 2,500 calories per day. If you eat more or less you will need to adjust these values.

Rapid changes in body weight are usually the result of changes in the amount of fluid the body retains or loses. Dieting initially causes weight loss from water or fluid loss. As your body adjusts to fewer calories, it begins using some of your fat stores for energy.

Table 18: Simple height/weight table

Height	Men	Women
First 5 feet	106 lbs.	100 lbs
For each inch over 5 feet	6 lbs.	5 lbs.

From this table, assuming that one pound of fat equals 3,500 calories, you can estimate the number of calories needed to either maintain, increase or decrease your weight. Fill in the form *Your own weight goals* on page 148.

This is only an estimate, so if you do need to change your body composition and amount of fat, the best method is to focus on the actual number of calories burned for your level of activity. You can estimate the number of calories needed

Table 19: Your own weight goals

Your Ideal Body Weight	_____ pounds
Pounds Over Ideal (Lose Weight)	lose _____ pounds
Pounds Under Ideal (Gain Weight)	gain _____ pounds

to maintain a particular weight with COPD, using the table *Estimate calories needed to maintain weight*.

Multiply your Ideal Weight by Calories for your Level of Activity to find Calories Needed Daily.

Table 20: Estimate calories needed to maintain weight

Level of activity	Exercise sessions each week	Calories per pound per day needed to maintain current weight
Inactive		11
Moderately Active	2-3	13
Active	4-5	15
Extremely Active	6-7	18
Inactive with weight loss		18

As fat contributes more calories than other sources, the present recommendation for normal adults is 30% of daily calories from fat. If you are at high risk for heart disease or need to lose body fat, then reduce fats to 25% or 20% of daily calories. If you need to gain weight, you can increase fat to as high as 50% a day, especially if you get short of breath from COPD when eating.

Using the two tables above, estimate the calories you need from fat. Use the examples in the tables below as reference.

1 Multiply your ideal weight in pounds by the number of calories you need, per pound (11, 13, 15, or 18).

2 Decide what percent of your calories must come from fat.

3 Multiply the number of calories you need per day by the percent to get the number of fat calories you need per day.

4 Then divide the result by 9 to find the number of grams of fat you need in a day. You now have a personal fat budget of _____ grams of fat per day.

For example, a woman needs 50%, 95 grams, or 858 calories of her total 1716 calories per day in fat, to gain weight. The number of calories contributed by fat and protein intake can be adjusted to meet her needs.

This calorie and fat intake should gradually reduce body fat and improve breathing as the individual loses weight.

Tips for Adjusting Your Weight

Losing weight

If you are overweight and need to reduce, an excellent strategy is to reduce fat in your diet. You can usually reduce fat without changing taste.

Table 21: Computing a personal nutritional budget for calories and fat

Ideal weight based on your height	106 pounds for 5 feet + ____ inches x 5 for a woman x 6 for a man	= _____ lbs ideal weight
Calories needed per pound	_____ lbs ideal weight x (11, 13, 15, or 18)	= _____ calories per day
Fat calories as % of food	_____ calories per day x (30, 40, or 50%)	= _____ calories of fat
Fat in grams	_____ calories of fat divided by 9	= _____ grams of fat per day

Table 22: Example of a nutritional budget for a female

67 years, 70 inches, 125 lbs, inactive, weight loss, dyspnea		
Ideal Weight	106 lbs. (for first 5 feet) + (5 lbs x 10 inches = 50 lbs.)	= 156 lbs ideal weight
Calories Needed	156 (Calculated ideal Weight) x 18 (calories needed per day)	= 1716 calories per day
Fat Calories	1716 calories per day x 50%	= 858 calories of fat
Grams of Fat	858 calories of fat / 9	= 95 grams of fat

Table 23: Example of a nutritional budget for a male

67 years, 70 inches, 225 lbs, with COPD, no weight loss, some dyspnea		
Ideal Weight	106 + 60	= 166 lbs ideal weight
Calories Needed	166 ideal weight x 11 calories per day	= 1826 calories per day
Fat Calories	1826 calories per day x 25%	= 456 Fat Calories
Grams of Fat	456 fat calories / 9	= 50 grams of fat

- Look for sources of fat in each recipe you use, and in your choices at restaurants.
- Look at the ingredients and at the means of preparation, such as cooking with butter and deep frying.
- Use only skim or 1% milk.
- Use one whole egg and whites for the others.
- Reduce butter or substitute margarine.
- Use low-fat cheeses, or reduce quantities.
- Avoid deep-fried foods.
- Prepare fried foods with Pam™ or another non-stick substitute.
- Use lemon juice and a bit of olive oil instead of mayonnaise or prepared salad dressings.

Gaining weight

If you are underweight, make a plan for eating and try to stick with it.

- Plan frequent small meals, or snacks, at definite times.
- Set up your schedule at your best times for breathing and medications.

- When possible, share the meal with someone.
- Plan variety.
- Use the services of Meals on Wheels if you are eligible to get more variety.
- Decide when the best time is for you to exercise each day, then reward yourself with a delicious snack.
- Pick out your favorite television show and plan to have a snack while watching.
- Play cards or dominoes while having a snack.

Preventing weight loss

Weight gain is easier if you can prevent worsening of your lung disease.

- Preventive measures such as immunizations against influenza, prompt treatment of any increase in wheezing and the treatment of infection are essential.
- During flu season or at times when there are respiratory illnesses in the community, try to avoid crowds.
- Almost all the epidemic infections like influenza, the "flu", are spread by droplets coughed or sneezed into the air. Ask friends and relatives to avoid visiting you if they have a cold or upper respiratory infection; an alternative is for them to wear a face mask, so that if they cough or sneeze the droplets will be caught by the mask. It may look silly and feel strange, but it may keep you from becoming ill. Keep a supply on hand just in case.
- Try to find the major reason for eating too little. Discuss with your doctor or a nutritionist, then use their advice to correct your eating habits.

Avoiding stress

Another important rule to prevent weight loss and illness is to avoid stress and take excitement in small doses. During holiday seasons in the fall and winter, many people are stressed by unusual numbers of visitors, some of whom expect large traditional meals, decorations and entertainment. Explain to the family that you would love to have the visit, but that they must assume the burden of decorating, cooking and cleaning. Give yourself plenty of rest time. Keep your bedroom off limits to visitors, as a quiet sanctuary. Ask your visitors to restore your house almost to normal before they leave so that the burden of cleaning, washing linens, scrubbing the bathrooms, is not yours. Be flexible about activities, but try to keep to your medicine schedule. Continue exercise; your grandchildren may enjoy stretching and doing low-impact aerobics with you.

Tips for Increasing Calories or Protein

To add calories:

- Add a teaspoon of butter or margarine to foods. It adds 45 calories. Mix it into hot foods such as soups, vegetables, mashed potatoes, cooked cereal and rice.
- Eat hot breads because you use more butter when it melts.
- Mayonnaise has 100 calories per tablespoon—almost twice as much as salad dressing. Use it on salads, with eggs, and in sandwiches.
- Peanut butter has a lot of protein and about 90 calories per tablespoon. Use on fruits, vegetables and other foods. Add to sandwiches with mayonnaise and cream cheese.
- Use honey for sweetening and as a snack.
- Use sour cream and yogurt on vegetables such as potatoes, beans, carrots and squash. Try them in gravies or as a dressing with sugar for fruit.

To add protein:

- Add skim milk powder to many of your recipes. This will add additional protein.
- Use fortified milk for cooking and drinking. Add milk powder to hot and cold cereals, scrambled eggs, soups, gravies and other baked recipes.
- Add meat to soups and casseroles.
- Add cheese to sauces, vegetables, soups, and casseroles.
- Use eggs liberally in a variety of dishes.
- Choose desserts that contain large amounts of eggs, such as rice and bread pudding, egg custard, angel food cake, brownies, and ice cream.
- Use peanut butter liberally.
- Eat fresh and prepared nuts as snacks.
- Eat more meat, fish and poultry.
- Drink milk shakes as snacks.

Diet and Medications

Some dietary problems may be caused by medications or interactions between medication and food. Certain foods may alter the effectiveness of a medicine, while certain medicines may alter your ability to use some nutrients in the foods you eat. Ask your doctor or hospital nutritionist for information and guidance about the medications you take and your body's ability to absorb nutrients.

9 Recipe for Living

In this chapter, Jo-Von writes of the things she has done to simplify, enjoy, and get on with her life. She gives useful advice on doing these things yourself. Her topics include:

- Support groups and how to get one going
- Keeping a journal
- Being sociable
- Enjoying life
- Simplifying daily activities.

Support Groups

Some people, particularly my family, seemed to expect me to carry on, as though nothing major had happened. I am sure this was partly my fault, because I never let them see my problems. I had always been very private. So they had unrealistic expectations of me. Other people appeared to think this was a passing weakness that would go away with positive thinking.

In Mark Doty's book *Heaven's Coast: A Memoir*, about his loss of his lover to AIDS, the line, "We trivialize pain if we regard it as a preventable condition the spirit need not suffer" leaped at me from the page. I reacted as though someone had hit me. I thought about how some people might blame me for getting sick like this, as though I could have avoided it. Or maybe they thought it was a punishment for evil deeds or bad thoughts. There is my pain and guilt for having smoked for many years, and an unsympathetic public is quick to say that we brought this illness upon ourselves.

For months after I arrived on Cape Cod, I searched for a lung-disease support group. I asked my doctor, respiratory therapist, oxygen provider, and pharmacist, read the papers, and other publications, but none existed.

I longed to be able to talk to others going through the same things. I longed for emotional support, and for understanding and empathy. With more than 30% of the Cape Cod population retired and senior citizens, it seemed peculiar that no such group existed, particularly as respiratory disease tends to afflict older people. I was sure there was need for a support group. The pulmonary specialists on the peninsula all had full, thriving practices. The numbers just had to be there.

I needed a forum where people with COPD could share their feelings and experiences, learn from each other and from experts in respiratory and pulmonary medicine. The people at the Chatham/Orleans Visiting Nurses Association told me that if I believed there was a need, then I should start one myself. So I did.

The empathy within a support group validates. Someone else feels as you do, someone understands what life is like with obstructive airway disease. I needed to search for those people to share their experiences. People who felt as I did would be my inspiration. They would help me define a lung support group.

Today, our meetings are full of people who share. There is a person next to me on oxygen too, and one across the room in a wheelchair, also on oxygen. There are people who have serious problems retaining carbon dioxide. There are people from many different age and ethnic groups. Some look sick, and some do not. But, none of us can breathe without effort. Every one grows short of breath with slight exertion, like walking in from the front door of the building to our meeting room.

Starting a Support Group

Although I didn't know if people would travel to belong to such a group, I decided on a Cape-wide project. I put together a plan. I imagined what sitting and talking with people who felt exactly as I did, who've felt the same fear and pain... precisely the same. The overriding feeling I had felt since diagnosis was isolation. It seemed to me that people shied away from me. Now I know that these reactions weren't aimed at me personally but were a general response to a reminder of their own mortality, especially if they were smokers.

A Mission Statement

I named my imaginary group "The Cape COPD Support Group" and wrote a mission statement for it:

"The Cape COPD Support Group's mission is to provide a forum to serve the needs of people with chronic obstructive pulmonary disease. It is our intent to educate ourselves about lung disease in order to learn how to better manage the illness, and to retain as much quality of life as possible. We seek input and data on new treatments and surgical procedures, as well as on exercise and rehabilitation, diet and attitude. And, most importantly, we wish to be able to share our feelings and information with those who have been struck down with the same illness."

My business background, my volunteer work, and my passion for the subject, helped me to set objectives, and get started. A strategic plan was not daunting. I had a strategic vision, and I knew what I wanted to accomplish.

Armed with a description of the new support group I set out to attract people to a first meeting through the local media. I wrote a brief blurb for two local newspapers and the local cable TV station community service announcements. I talked to people I saw with oxygen equipment, or who were obviously having difficulty breathing. Some people, especially spouses, approached me as I was visible where many people were too embarrassed to take their portable oxygen public. I was not self-conscious anymore, very active, and could be seen all over the Outer Cape wearing my oxygen cannula and toting my portable unit from a shoulder strap.

The first meeting took place at my home, and four people showed up. One had to leave immediately as I had two cats in the house, and she was allergic. We agreed we needed a support group, and I contacted the Orleans Council on Aging to see if we could hold meetings at the Orleans Senior Center. This fine facility has been our meeting place now for more than seven years.

Finding a Sponsor

After a few meetings, I contacted the Southeastern branch of The American Lung Association of Massachusetts to see if they would become our sponsor and give us more credibility. They would, and they did. They provided us with booklets on COPD, emphysema, asthma and on breathing exercises. And they agreed to reimburse us for the cost of postage to mail out meeting announcements, which later became our monthly newsletter. In promotion and identification of our group, we state that we are sponsored by the The American Lung Association.

Meetings

Our first few meetings were based on the booklets provided by the ALA. They were get-acquainted meetings, that lasted two hours on the second Wednesday of each month, from 2 to 4 in the afternoon. We began to share our feelings and experiences, tentatively at first. Within a few months, between word of mouth and continuing public relations, we had about 16 members, and many came to the meetings with a spouse or caregiver. Our numbers grew rapidly, as did our rapport and friendship. Seven years later, the Cape COPD Support Group has 125 loyal, active, involved members, who are the bravest, most courageous people I know.

We decided early to alternate our monthly meetings between qualified speakers and discussion groups. I believe that it has helped keep our group as interested and lively as it is. One month we have speakers on a range of subjects, the next month round-table discussions among ourselves, where each member is invited to speak, if they choose.

Speakers

A lot of work is involved in contacting potential speakers, but it has been rewarding and we have had no trouble signing up good speakers. Cape Cod Hospital's Community Affairs Department has helped us, and we have had excellent talks on COPD by leading pulmonologists, Dr. Mohr has made five appearances over the years, and we've benefited from the teachings of respiratory therapists on breathing exercises. Here are a few of the subjects and guest speakers we have hosted:

- Pulmonary Specialists
- Respiratory Therapists
- Nutrition Experts
- Asthma/Allergy Specialist
- Paramedic/EMTs on Emergency Procedures
- Psychologists
- Pharmacists
- Physical Rehabilitation Specialists or Exercise Physiologist
- Meditation Instructors
- Book Reviews on Related Health Issue Publications
- T'ai Chi Exercise Classes

- Managing Daily Living
- Stress Management
- Pulmonary rehabilitation nurses.

Discussion Group Sessions

In the discussion groups, every person can speak briefly about their concerns or issues. They may tell the group a bit about their own illness or ask questions. We have never found ourselves at a loss for words. Rather, we run out of time. Many people have no one else to talk to about lung disease, or about their problems. Lots of them live alone, as I do, or with family members who don't understand or even try to know what they are going through. Once our members realize that they are free to say whatever they feel, and to express their emotions in an environment of total understanding, the flood gates open.

We share a great deal of vital and helpful information. For example, I'd had a recurring problem of sensitivity and soreness including nose bleeds and crusty sores caused by continuous use of oxygen. I'd been fighting this problem for a couple of years. I tried Mentholatum in my nose, but one member told me that this was quite dangerous, that glycerine-based salve should never be mixed with oxygen. He told me about a water-soluble salve, Ayr, available at pharmacies, to counteract dryness of oxygen use.

I have found that our support group members open up within these sessions, expressing deeply hidden feelings and frustrations. The atmosphere is caring and sharing; you can feel the empathy in the room. Sometimes eyes fill with tears. Many times there's laughter.

For some of our members, getting dressed and out is a real effort, so we try to make their two hours with us as physically comfortable as possible. We are comfortable when we can lean our arms on a table for breathing support, so we set up our meetings in chairs around long tables, arranged in a U-shape, for maximum comfort and good eye contact. Coffee is provided at each meeting, even during the summer, because we've learned that a hot beverage helps open up clogged airways.

Dues

There were initially no dues, but we did accept contributions. Now, with such a large membership, we ask for a contribution of $24 yearly from each member, if they can afford it. This helps us reimburse the Orleans Senior Center for coffee they prepare for each meeting, and helps with operating expenses like printing envelopes and mailing newsletters.

Committees

Because many people are terminally ill with COPD and house-bound, we formed a committee to visit home or hospital. Committees are great for projects like this, allowing members to participate as fully as they wish. Aside from the Outreach Committee, we have:

- An Advisory Panel to help plan programs, guest speakers and projects
- A Telephone Committee
- A Fire Department Information Committee.
- A committee to work on the Medicare oxygen cuts.

On the Fire Department Information Project a volunteer member from each village collects data on every support group member for the database of the Fire Department of each town. Whenever an emergency call goes to a Fire Department from a member's house, important information is available on the way to the address. This can save lives. We have found the fire chiefs very cooperative about using this information.

The data we provide is:

- Person's name
- Address and phone
- State of health
- Medications and dosages
- Allergies
- Use of supplemental oxygen and the liter flow
- Name and phone number of pulmonary doctor
- Next-of-kin information
- Complications such as heart problems, hypertension or diabetes, and their prescribed treatment.

The Fire Department or Emergency Service puts the patient information into their database for instant access so that EMTs can call up critical information on the way. A call to 911 provides all of this information, so that these first responders know what to expect and how to begin treatment, even if the person is too ill to speak to them or to the 911 operator.

Socials and Friendships

We plan two social events for the entire group during the year. A Summer Covered Dish Social or Cookout is at the home of a member. A Christmas Gala coincides with our December meeting. Both occasions are gatherings of friends, and of people who share with them.

Another offshoot of our support group is a group of the wives who have formed a mini-support-group for caregivers, meeting for lunch several times a month. This provides a warm and caring forum for those who care for those with COPD, and who frequently suffer as much from the effects of this illness as we do.

Publicity

Our meeting notices are in community-service bulletins all over the Cape, in all media. Guest speakers and their topics are provided, a little information about the group, and date, time, and place. I usually fax the information to the media. We have a constant stream of guests and new members from all 16 villages on Cape Cod, and from as far away as New Bedford and Provincetown. Two stories about our group in the local papers generated a lot of interest in our meetings, and resulted in more members.

Newsletters

After only a few meetings, we realized that a newsletter would be an excellent way of reaching our members to remind them of meetings, and to promote guest speakers. Some people are too sick to attend meetings and quite a few go to warmer climates during the winter, so the newsletter keeps us in touch with each other. It also provides information about our support group to doctors and various health care professionals and organizations. Referrals from doctors have become a good source of new members for us.

The Cape COPD Newsletter gives news of our members, welcomes new ones, mourns the passing of some, reprints articles and editorials of interest, and encourages people to live life to the fullest. One member, Donna B. MacDonald, is a published author and writes a column, "Donna's Department" for each issue. Donna has bronchiectasis, and her columns are delightful, full of spunk and life, encouragement and information. Occasionally we print vignettes about our members.

Our newsletter goes out to about 250 people, 125 members and the rest to doctors, health care organizations, and other interested parties, like Councils on Aging, local VNAs, and Cape Cod Hospital. We include all doctors who treat our members, to help personalize people to their doctors. And it certainly results in a steady stream of referrals for membership.

I write the newsletter, then photocopy it onto three double-sided pages, or have it printed and collated. The ALA reimburses us for postage and some photocopies. I generate the mailing labels on my computer. Members of our support group stuff, seal and label the envelopes.

Brochure

One of our best investments has been production of a brochure about the Cape COPD Support Group. The American Lung Association paid for printing, but the rest of it was prepared camera-ready on my computer. The brochure is 8 1/2" x 11", folded twice to fit into a standard #10 envelope. That format gives six panels of information.

We describe ourselves as "A caring, sharing support system for people with chronic obstructive pulmonary disease." We give our mission statement, invite folks to meetings, and offer to send our newsletter. We provide brochures to pulmonary specialists, councils on aging, senior centers, Visiting Nurse Associations, and to companies providing oxygen services for distribution to interested people.

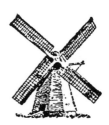

Cape C.O.P.D. Support Group

A Caring, Sharing Support System
for People with
Chronic Obstructive Pulmonary Disease.

The Cape C.O.P.D. Support Group is a non-profit organization that is sponsored by the Southeastern Branch of The American Lung Association of Massachusetts.

Our mission is to learn as much as possible about the illnesses that we suffer, in order to be able to better manage our lives, and to retain as much *quality of life* as we can.

We seek to provide a forum for C.O.P.D. patients to be able to talk among ourselves with other people who truly understand the perspective of the disease, and to encourage the pushing of boundaries and expression of feelings.

The Cape COPD Research Library

A new and especially promising project is our Cape COPD Research Library, whose purpose is to provide our members and Newsletter subscribers with up-to-date research and information on obstructive lung disease and related issues. We have compiled information (much of it from the Internet) on COPD, medications, experimental surgeries and treatments, symptoms and other topics. Members of our support group are provided with a list of subjects to choose from, to receive information. Or they add a subject.

Donna and her mother, Ruth, prepare a package to send out in response to inquiries. If no information is on file, they will research the subject on the Internet and send what they find. There is no charge to members for this service. At this time we charge non-members a minimal fee to cover postage, usually $3 per subject.

We believe this will prove to be an important resource on COPD for people who may not have computer access or be able to conduct their own research.

Keeping it Going

Keeping a support group going is not easy. It takes lots of planning to keep members interested and involved, and at least in New England, to get people to participate. We have between 30 and 50 people at a meeting, and I have learned the hard way that you can't please everybody, all the time. Some will think the room too cold, others too warm. Some will like the guest speaker, and some will not. Some may vehemently disagree with the speaker. Some members may be disagreeable, and some even rude. But it is never a personal attack, just folks who know how to speak their minds. If things get a little loud or out of hand, we have a desk bell to get everyone to settle back down and focus on the speaker. The trick with these minor upheavals is to not take them personally. Each member of our group now feels comfortable enough with the others to be able to speak directly and honestly about their feelings, and they do.

The more I give to this group the more I receive. Active participation in a support group has been a very positive experience for me, as I am sure it has been for others. I've learned a lot about the illness, as we have educated ourselves about lung disease. Since COPD is still relatively unknown by the general public, we've also accomplished a good bit of education outside our world through our publicity efforts.

Figure 38   At a meeting of the Cape Cod COPD Support Group

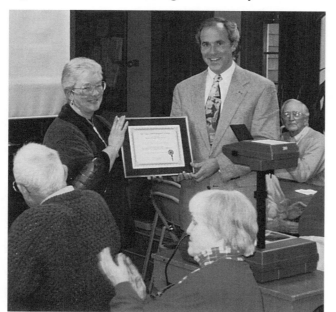

Jo-Von Tucker presenting an award to Dr. Paul Sklarew, M.D., in recognition of his generous efforts on behalf of the Cape COPD Support Group. Photo ©1998 Francis Birch

Checklist for Starting a Support Group

1 Name your group.
2 Write a mission statement, and/or objectives.
3 Why a group.
4 What the group will do.
5 What the group will achieve.
6 Decide the first meeting place, date, and time.
7 Publicize the first meeting: doctors' offices, hospitals, media, through groups, in person.
8 Encourage word of mouth.
9 Hold meetings.
10 Get a sponsor.
11 Plan activities and projects.
12 Invite speakers.
13 Share.

Other Kinds of Support

I've observed the reluctance of some members of my family to accept the reality of my illness, and its ramifications. It seems very difficult for them to know the details of the diagnosis, or to understand the stress and strain of having to make the required lifestyle adjustments just to carry on.

If you are faced with chronic illness as a patient, it is best to grasp quickly the struggles that your loved ones are going through, too. Best to understand that it is not possible for them to relate to your battle with disease or illness as you would like them to. Easier on everyone if you develop a quiet strength and reserve on your own, along with infinite patience in helping those around you absorb the condition and the prognosis.

You'll find ways to help educate your family and friends about your illness, maybe in bits and bytes. It seems to me that digestion of the facts is easier in small quantities. If you pay close attention to their feelings, as well as to your own, you'll be able to judge their need for information. If you try to give too many details at one time, you run the risk of having them back away from you. Don't resent them for it, it's a natural flight response to bad news.

While I recommend a gradual sharing of facts and information about your chronic illness, I am not suggesting that you deceive anyone by misleading or Pollyanna reactions to questions. Just look for ways to truthfully let them know how you are, without gory details or ill-timed specifics. There seems to be a separate culture for dealing with sick people, or for patients to deal with their loved ones. It should be one based on truth and caring, on both sides.

All of these are reasons why you'll find great strength and solace from a support group. These are people who know exactly how you feel. They have fought the same battles, felt the same emotions, raged at the same demons. They, more than anyone else in your life, will be able to share your fears, hear about your wins and your losses, and exult over your triumphs, just as they grieve over your sorrows. Participation in a good support group will provide you with an outlet for self-expression, and an opportunity to help others as much as they can help you.

There is no need to wage your war alone.

The Family Support System

The closest and most important part of a COPD patient's entire system of support is the family. Spouses, siblings, sons and daughters are the people most affected by illness, other than the patient. They may be called upon to implement changes in their lives, just as you will. They will surely be relied upon more heavily as physical accomplishments become more difficult and limited. And usually they are the first to feel the reverberations of your anguish and rage.

Family will also be most able to provide a firm foundation of love, care and concern for you. In order to best accomplish this, they need to learn as much as possible about lung disease, and about its effects. This knowledge will help them as they help you deal with each exacerbation, with every lung infection, and with each mood swing of your drastically altered life.

Family members need to be able to walk the fine line between helping you and co-dependency. It will be important to your self-esteem and emotional well-being for caregivers to recognize when help is needed, not to simply take over and do everything when you are increasingly disabled.

Another fine line is trying to provide encouragement for you, without seeming to be uncaring or unconcerned. Family members can play an important role in building your self-confidence. Family can provide hope and positive feedback when you are sorely in need of both to help you get through the most difficult times.

To the Caregiver

If you are a caregiver for a lung patient, I congratulate you for "already being there" for your affected person by reading this book. You are interested enough in helping to have started your own search for knowledge. There are many other ways you can provide the necessary support system, little ways and big ways. Whether it's a smile and a hug, or accompanying the person to a doctor's appointment, your contributions are important. Your emotional support will go a long way toward keeping your loved one vital, involved, active and alive.

Throughout this book, we encourage people to take an active and responsible role in management of their illness. In order for them to do so, they need your help. Please continue to be there for them, and to be a part of their ongoing battle with chronic obstructive pulmonary disease. You can help them find the courage to go on.

Keeping Your Own Library

Having your own modest library can be extremely helpful.

I have referred to my own library on obstructive airway disease hundreds of times over the last ten years, and know that I will continue to rely on it for helpful tips and important issues. Each time I get sick with a lung infection or a passing virus, I find myself delving into my library for anything relevant, something to help me fight the illness. And I often find something, such as a reminder about the importance of nutrition in battling life-threatening illnesses, or how helpful a room humidifier can be during the dry heat of winter.

Keeping a Journal

Keeping a journal serves several purposes:

- It gives you something to do, and provides continuity. Try to write a little every day. You may be surprised at how easy it is.
- You can be as philosophical as you like, as whimsical as you please, as entertaining or as mundane as you choose. You can whine if you need to. No one is there to pass judgment.
- You can express your innermost feelings. No one can be hurt or angered by what you write, and self-expression can ward off depression. It allows you to vent. Let it flow.
- Document your battle with chronic illness. You'll be able to flip through the pages later and see your progress. This can provide wonderful encouragement.
- Write about pleasant times and memories to enjoy again later.
- You can include sketches and memorabilia.

You may find that keeping a journal is something you are good at. Lots of writers start this way. See excerpts from Jo-Von's journals in *Journal Samples* on page 213.

Being Sociable

It has been said that people with COPD seem to just fade away. People may make the easiest choice of surrendering to the illness, waiting at home for the inevitable, rather than fighting. This is true even for people who were quite social, before illness. Whether this stems from embarrassment caused by people gawking at oxygen equipment, or lack of energy is unclear. It does take an enormous amount of energy to be sociable, whether meeting friends for dinner, or having folks over for bridge.

Just a few years ago, people with emphysema and other lung disorders were confined to bed rest at home, with their oxygen tanks. Now, thanks to portable oxygen equipment, relative freedom of movement is possible.

It is healthier to live life to its fullest, but encouragement may be needed to get out and about. Family members can play an important role as a staunch support system, getting you out for a drive, or encouraging you to keep active in community affairs. Active involvement in a support group may develop new friendships with people who are in the same situation. This can add a whole new dimension for you and your spouse or partner. Even though it takes effort, it is energy well spent.

My daughter is great about encouraging me to attend my granddaughter's soccer games. It wears me out to trudge across the field to the bleachers, dragging my portable oxygen tank, but I'm always glad I made the effort to see Shelby in action. We go to movies together, are together on all holidays, and occasionally take turns cooking dinner for each other.

I am lucky to live where I do, because Cape Cod has a never-ending procession of festivals, arts and crafts shows, and neat places to go and things to do.

Interests and hobbies can be lifelines for the chronically ill. Many interests and activities can be paced so as not to overexert.

I can no longer crawl on my belly to get dramatic shots of giraffes in East Africa, but I can still take extraordinary shots of the flora and fauna of Cape Cod. I even give speeches at conferences. I still command the respect I had before appearing with a portable oxygen tank. I am a bit breathless when I arrive at the podium, but recover quickly.

Outings are a great way to socialize and with the freedom provided by a portable liquid oxygen unit you can have six or more hours away from home. In the Northeast, there are day trips to casinos for a few enjoyable hours of playing blackjack or pulling handles on the one-arm bandits. There are lectures and book signings, poetry readings, museums, and art galleries, movies, antique shops and hundreds of other things to enjoy.

Do things with other people. Call members of your support group to see if they'd like to go with you to an event. Self-esteem soars as you find common interests, and days pass more pleasantly and faster.

Try correspondence. Correspondence is a terrific activity. It invites a response, and it can be generated at your convenience, anytime you have a few minutes. You can enjoy receiving mail from people all over the country or the world. Get on electronic mail if you have a computer, or stock your desk with writing materials: your favorite stationery, plenty of stamps and pens, and pictures to share. You can stock up on an assortment of cards: birthday, anniversary, thinking-of-you. If you have a computer and are on the internet, there are even websites to send animated greeting cards. The selections today are fabulous, with very specific and personal messages to choose from. And a stash of thank-you cards is handy for all those really nice things that people do for you.

Most people enjoy children. Whether grandchildren or children from your neighborhood, there is something brightening about spending time with babies and kids, playing as they do, and enjoying their flights of imagination and creativity. The world of children is simpler than the adult world, and children are always ready to invite you there, if only for a little while. It's a great escape from concerns and stresses. Offer to read a book or a story to a child, and just watch the face light up.

The thing to remember when planning visits with children and grandchildren is conserving energy. Be careful not to overdo. Don't allow your visit to deteriorate into exhaustion and short temper. Grown-up children can help by not expecting visits with beloved grandchildren to become extended baby-sitting.

Dealing with Strangers

The downside of being in public with oxygen gear is dealing with people who stare or make rude remarks.

I remember how easily upset I was when first adjusting to supplemental oxygen. Strangers in elevators asked me what was wrong. I didn't want to explain about my condition to strangers, and I was offended by their rudeness. I suspected that people who behaved like this thought that we are contagious, and that they may be exposed.

After nearly ten years, I've learned to ignore rudeness, and am much better about not getting upset. The incidents still happen, but I deal with them better. And I refuse to let such episodes keep me from doing whatever I want. If I feel compelled, I answer questions with a brief statement that I have chronic obstructive pulmonary disease, which is not contagious. This is usually enough.

Some people simply smile directly at someone who is staring, and say "Hello." This can even lead to interesting new acquaintances, and usually helps to educate the public.

Enjoying Life

Ask yourself what joy means to you. Is it the sound of birds singing? Is it a relationship? Do memories of good times, or tastes or feelings conjure happy memories? Good times are the easiest to remember. Living with a chronic illness means that every day, even the good ones, will be filled with negatives. So it is imperative to live in the moment, finding joy, happiness, comfort, and love where and when we can. But we can create those moments too, not just expect them to land in our laps.

Force yourself to go regularly in search of good times. Positive feelings and memories of happy experiences will go a long way toward overcoming the negative effects of illness. And more: anticipation helps you to face each day, to forget pain and suffering for a while. Anticipation makes you nicer to be around, gives you a good reason to get up and out each day, and to find things that make you happy.

Your search for joy

Your mind can transport you to a different place with pleasant, positive images even while experiencing pain. You need to focus and concentrate. Think of a favorite place, a private place you love. See it, smell it, hear it, taste it, touch it. You can go there by visualizing and meditating.

JoAnn LeMaistre, in her book, *After the Diagnosis*, advises us to look for moments that can be framed, that can be used on days when life is hard. Take inventory, both past and present, to identify moments of sheer happiness that you can write about and think of later. Make a list of the things you were doing at the time that resulted in happiness. Keep this list close by. Use it to remind yourself of the things that bring you pleasure. You can subdivide your list into things for your good, active days, and things better saved for times when you are house bound. Then, do them.

Activities

For Less Active Days

Jo-Von's list may stimulate your own.

- Jigsaw puzzles, the really complicated, intricate ones with no edge pieces
- Needlepoint
- Reading
- Corresponding with friends and family
- Working on photo albums
- Writing a journal, or reading previous entries and remembering
- Watching birds around feeders
- On a warm day, sitting for a while with your face turned to the sun
- A cup of jasmine tea on a rainy day
- Playing cards or Backgammon
- Solitaire
- Trying out new recipes
- Telephoning friends
- Favorite magazines
- Coloring with fine point markers in a grown-up coloring book
- Sculpting with modeling clay
- Watching old, classic movies, or any suspense thriller
- Making notecards with rubber stamps and ink pads
- Going for a drive, parking, and looking at the ocean or any view
- Scrabble
- Listening to music
- Writing poetry
- Remembering beloved family members.

For Active Days

- Photography
- Gardening
- Walks with a pet
- Movies
- Shopping
- Entertaining friends or family with homecooked meals
- Dinner at a favorite restaurant
- Croquet

- Tree swings
- Travel
- Museums
- Art galleries
- Whale watching trips
- Bird watching
- Visiting with grandchildren
- Picnics
- Exploring backroads.

Live fully in the moment. All of these activities and interests provide opportunities to create a rich tapestry of memories. There are many experiences during the course of each day that can bring you delight, spontaneous things like social exchanges with people around you, things you see and hear. Living fully in the moment means really paying attention as things happen. You can be just as joyful at dewdrops on a lily as experiencing a dramatic rain-and-thunder storm.

Joy is an elusive emotion, but one worth pursuing and storing. You can train yourself to be aware of good things, and to accentuate the positive. It may need some extra discipline, and some practice, but for people with chronic illness, concentrating on the positive should be a requirement. If there is not enough joy and happiness in your life, go find some. Stock up on good memories until your mental library is bulging. Reach for the good times, create an oasis of cool waters and waving palm trees in the middle of your desert.

On the other hand, you cannot force this. You have to have an instinct for survival, and be willing to commit to learning to live in the moment. To quote again from *After the Diagnosis*, "Part of your goal is to be as emotionally able-hearted as possible, despite your physical limitations."

Like JoAnn LeMaistre, I believe that people can creatively adapt and use their internal powers of wholeness (the sense of being emotionally intact) to reduce physical limitations. Look outward to get through pain and loss, and to re-establish quality of life. Look inward to find your strengths and courage.

Many good books on meditation and visualization are available in your library or bookstore.

Simplifying Daily Activities

Maybe you look at restrictions dictated by lung disease as barriers. My nature is to push at boundaries to see what I can get away with. I certainly advocate doing so with COPD. Pushing the barriers means staying busy, enjoying the things that I can do, and constantly trying to do a little more.   *JVT*

Independence is extremely important. It promotes well-being and dignity. Push the boundaries, try to achieve the maximum, and each accomplishment becomes a victory. No one can feel really good about sitting back and expecting others to wait on them like servants. It is much healthier to feel capable of taking care of your own necessities for living. Compromises must be made, but do as much for yourself as possible, for both the rehabilitation and the independence.

Shopping for Groceries

Grocery stores and super markets today are huge, sprawling things with departments like delis, bakeries, banks and pharmacies, even gardening and flower centers. This is both good and bad news: great because you can one-stop-shop for most needs, not so great because it is an exhausting trip.

As people with COPD suffer from extreme fatigue most of the time, akin to a normal, healthy person who has just run 10 miles, any exertion or exercise means even deeper fatigue. So the solution for grocery shopping can be provided by electric carts. They are terrific for disabled people and the elderly. If your local mall or supermarket, or grocery store does not provide such a service for the handicapped, put in a request, or find a chain that does.

I found it a little embarrassing riding in the electric shopping cart at first, but got over that quickly when I realized how helpful the cart was, making it possible for me to shop. One problem for me is that the electric cart moves at a snail's pace, way too slow for my taste. I would prefer a little more speed so I can get through the dreaded chore faster. But then, having seen how some of my neighbors drive cars, perhaps the slow speed of the carts is a good thing. I don't want to be run down in Aisle 3 by a cart at high speed as I reach for the spaghetti sauce.

Another problem is that occasionally the store manager or staff forget to plug in the carts for recharging, resulting in carts with dead or fading batteries. It really isn't fun to get half-way finished shopping, only to have my chariot chug to a stop at the far end of the store. Then I must walk back up front to see if the other cart is available and functional, driving it to where I left the loaded carcass of my previous transportation, and then unloading into the new vehicle's basket. The long walk to the front of the store is enough to rob me of breath, and the aerobic impact of using my arms to unload and reload the new cart leaves me drained, and cursing quietly.

You may have more trouble doing activities with arms than with legs, because you take blood flow and oxygen away from the breathing muscles when you use your arms. Regularly exercising your arms may help. Ask your doctor. *RC, BN, JVT*

House Cleaning

The two most difficult house-cleaning chores are making the bed and vacuuming.

Making up the bed each morning need not be one of your priorities. You may be just as happy if your bed is neatly straightened with the covers pulled up, not with a spread and toss pillows anchored firmly in position, requiring too much effort. No one is going to come from *Architectural Digest* or *House Beautiful* to photograph your bedroom each day. And there are no Bedroom Police.

I do formally make the bed if I am expecting company or house guests. But that puts bed making in the "special occasion only" category. I have found that the pleasure of slipping between the bed covers each night is not at all diminished if that bed hasn't spent its day in military conformity. Of course, I live alone and spend my days at work, so there's no one around to do bed checks on me.

Vacuuming is hard because it involves repeated motions of unsupported arms, becomes an aerobic exercise, and puts extra strain on already taxed heart and lungs. And the dust raised by such activity can be harmful to damaged lungs. It does help to wear a surgical mask for sweeping, dusting or vacuuming, to filter out most of the pollen and dirt raised by cleaning activity. If you can afford the service, have a cleaning person for a few hours every so often to do the heavier cleaning chores.

It would be much better if I could have help come more frequently, or for longer sessions, but cleaning help is very expensive on the Cape, and I cannot afford more services than those for which I am already committed. Days between the visits I deal with on my own. That includes regular dusting and cleaning which I don't like but I do, because the alternative is living in a dusty, dirty house.

Housework is a lot easier in a house all on one level. It is difficult to maneuver stairs to and from the basement to bring in groceries, do the laundry, or work in the yard in a multi-level house or apartment.

Laundry

With only one person in my household, laundry can be accomplished in a couple of loads. The hard part in my old house was the steep basement stairs carrying laundry baskets of clothing and linens. I had to do without supplemental oxygen, because I couldn't carry the portable unit and a laundry basket. The tubing to my stationary tank was not long enough to reach down the stairs and across the basement floor to the washing machine and dryer. Even carrying the basket was hazardous, so I maneuvered those monster stairs very carefully. Laundry is a breeze now, as the machines are just around the corner from the kitchen, same level.

Think about ways to ease the physical load of your daily activities. You may have to move to a more-efficient or smaller place.   *RC*

Meal Planning and Preparation

To avoid spending a lot of time cooking, I've devised a system that works pretty well for me all week long. If, however, you are prescribed oxygen for continuous use, extra care must be taken for the sake of safety. If you have a gas stove, for example, you may need to get another type of stove that is safe to use in the presence of oxygen.

WARNING: **Stay at least eight (8) feet away from an open flame while using oxygen. Do not use oxygen while cooking with an open flame such as gas appliances, or gas or charcoal-fired barbecue.**

WARNING: **Ask your home care equipment provider or your doctor if it is safe for you to cook with an electric stove or a microwave oven while using your oxygen.**

Dinners

I'm always pretty tired by evening, so the prospect of a shortcut is appealing.

- On the weekend I bake a small chicken or a roast with vegetables, or cook a small ham or pork roast. Then, for at least a couple of days, I enjoy a simple warm-up meal when I get home in the evenings.

- Alternate with fish, or shrimp, or even a steak. This takes the hassle out of making evening meals, including minimal kitchen duty.

- Baking a potato for dinner? Wrap two Irish or sweet potatoes in foil and cook them in the oven at the same time. One can be warmed up for dinner the next evening. Just refrigerate the extra potato (in its foil jacket) after it has cooled.

Breakfasts

Breakfast, the meal that is important for giving you the right start on your day, can be easily prepared and is rich with opportunity for diversity. With COPD you often have trouble in the mornings, and may be exhausted from showering, or from trying to cough up mucous. In order to save energy and still get nourishment, learn and practice some shortcuts:

- Pre-section your grapefruit the night before. Wrap the sectioned grapefruit halves in Saran™ wrap and refrigerate overnight.

- Prepare the coffee maker before you turn in at night. Fill the filter and add water to the reservoir. All you'll have to do in the morning is push the start button. Add a dash of ground cinnamon to your coffee. It mellows the coffee and eliminates acrid oils from the coffee beans.

- Set your place setting the previous night. Use a place mat for easy clean-up.

- Plan your breakfast menus for a week at a time, including fruit juice for each day. Apple, cranberry, orange, tomato, pineapple and grapefruit juices will provide a variety of taste and essential vitamins and minerals. Note: Grapefruit juice can alter the effect of certain medications. Check with your pharmacist to be safe.

- Crispy bacon blotted with a paper towel, once or twice a week, adds protein, niacin and "good" carbohydrates to your diet. The microwave bacon products such as Hormel, are delicious, easy to cook, and turn out crispy with most of the fat cooked out.

- Sprinkle a handful of fresh cranberries into your oatmeal as it cooks, for a healthy and different taste.

- Use whole-grain cereals with 2% milk and a sliced banana once or more during the week.

- Stew your own apricot jam in a small pan with a little water and lemon juice added to dried apricots. It makes a great spread for your buttered 7-grain toast slices.

- Cook eggs: fry them in a little Pam™, or scramble them with a little milk, add grated cheese. Poach 'em, hard-boil 'em, coddle or soft boil 'em. And forget about the scare several years ago about eggs and cholesterol that has since been rescinded.

Lunches

You can make quick work of lunch. Plan each week, and select dishes that are to your liking but don't require a lot of cooking or peeling:

- Make tuna fish or chicken salad for several days use.

- Serve as a sandwich, with slices of fresh avocado, or as a salad with crackers and fruit. Avocados are rich in potassium.

- In cold weather, hot soups are nourishing and easy.

- If you are hard-boiling eggs for chicken or tuna salad, add a couple extra to enjoy at night with your dinner.

- Stock your freezer with leftover serving portions of chili, soups, roasts, vegetables, casseroles... and bring them out for enjoyment whenever you feel less like cooking.

Snacks

For snacks between meals:

- •Help yourself to a handful of shelled walnuts, or to half a dozen dried apricots.
- •Yogurt makes a good mid-day or mid-afternoon snack, and helps to build protection against bacterial stomach and intestinal infections.
- •Avoid processed sugar snacks that will spike your blood sugars, only to have them fall drastically in short order.
- •Drink plenty of fluids, especially water, all during the day.

Working in the Garden, and Other Yard Work

If you have a garden your yardwork will probably be somewhat curtailed, so choose your priorities carefully. You may not be able to dig and do heavy planting, but you can enjoy planning and overseeing, and reaping the rewards.

I dearly love to work in my flower gardens and tinker around with plantings in my yard, so it upsets me that I can't do as much yard work as I would like. Even carrying my portable oxygen tank with me is not enough help for me to be able to weed and plant and prune. So I've compromised by hiring someone to mow the lawn and occasionally to clean the flower beds. I try to work in the garden for little parcels of time, concentrating on small areas, and have been fairly successful with large flowering pots for the deck, especially if I can get things set up for working in one location. Even so, I have to have help in major weeding and planting projects.

I've also discovered the pleasure of raising tomato plants on my deck, which faces West and gets lots of direct sun. It's wonderful to enjoy the sweet, bright red, vine-ripened tomatoes from my own plants. This is a totally manageable project that requires little more than consistent watering and feeding, with occasional pinching back, and training and tying vines to support stakes. What a joy. I'm planning to expand my tomato-growing activities with different kinds of tomatoes and more of them.

Plan your garden spots so that you can see them from all your windows, even if you are sick in bed. Use indoor plants and flowers to brighten your home and sweeten the air, with large green leafy plants like marginatas and corn plants to help purify the oxygen in a room.

Watering your gardening projects is something you can accomplish on your own with a garden hose, or more than one at different locations.

I've set up one long hose for use at the front of the house, and another one for use on the side and back. It's a bit like having one stationery liquid oxygen tank at home, and another one set up at my office.

Entertaining Guests

It really is advisable to establish that guests help themselves, rather than having them sit back and let you bring things to them. Find ways to make them feel comfortable with this.

I enjoy entertaining friends and family, whether it is for a meal or as a houseguest for several days. Since I live alone, I find the company something to look forward to. With limitations on my physical activities I have learned to politely inform my guests before they arrive that I cannot wait on them, and that they will have the run and hospitality of my home, but will have to do many things for themselves. I have the pantry and fridge fully stocked with groceries and drinks, and fresh linens and towels in the linen closet.

After guests are settled in, I ask if they would like a drink, and then show them the liquor cabinet. They seem to quickly grasp that they are on their own for bartending.

In my home, guests are expected to make their own beds, and to pick up after themselves. Thoughtful and considerate house guests are invited back again and again, and are welcome to call with a request for a stopover anytime. But guests who abuse my hospitality or take advantage of me will find my Cape Cod house "all booked up" the next time they try to arrange a stay.

I try to cook for my guests when I feel like it, because it is something I love doing, but I am not shy about asking for help setting the table, or clearing after the meal. If I am not feeling well we dine out. Or, lucky me, I can bring a fresh Lobster Clambake home with me, to my guests delight. It is such an easy way to entertain, and just requires about half an hour of steaming in beer to turn out perfectly. I get to enjoy the feast as much as my guests do.

It is important that your prospective guests understand fully the limitations that you have with obstructive lung disease. If you are embarrassed to tell them yourself, send for the very informative pamphlet, *Sick Lungs Don't Show*, from The American Lung Association of Hennepin County. This is an amazing little folder, written and sponsored by the Family Support Group of the ALA/Hennepin County, in Minneapolis, Minnesota. It contains brief but important information about living with chronic lung disease, physically, socially and emotionally.

I keep a copy of *Sick Lungs Don't Show* on the night stand in my guest bedroom, because sometimes I am too timid or even embarrassed to explain to my house guests, particularly if they are not old friends or relatives. I know that my guests read it, and that it helps them to understand the impact of illness on my life.

Even though I am on supplemental oxygen, attached by tubing to an oxygen cylinder, people tend to forget about the problem or become inured to seeing the oxygen cannula on my face. At home I have very long lengths of tubing attached to the stationary liquid oxygen. It has become a joke among my house guests that they always know where to find me by following the trail of plastic tubing.

Driving

I take great pleasure in being able to drive my own car wherever I wish. I have even taken some relatively long trips to Maine and Vermont, and to Connecticut, and have been very comfortable doing so. I most enjoy the time I am able to spend here on the Cape by the ocean, transported by my trusty Jeep Cherokee, just sitting and watching the tides or the spectacular sunsets with my dog beside me. I can't run and play on the beach anymore, but I sure do enjoy being there. It's the most restorative thing I do on a regular basis. For me, the sounds of the waves, the smell of the ocean air, the feel of the wind on my face and the sun's warmth on the top of my head—I am as joyful as the gulls as they wheel and glide in the air, simply enjoying their element. Okay, my wheeling and gliding days are over, but I've found enormous comfort in just being there.

These times of just being by the water have become my way of recharging my inner batteries. I try to spend a little time each morning on the way to work, and each evening on my way home, observing/resting/thinking/not-thinking by the grey-blue waters of Cape Cod Bay or Rock Harbor where I can watch "The Rock Harbor bandits", otherwise known as the charter fishing fleet, come in bearing flags that brag of their catch.

Other Activities

For every thing that you can no longer do, there are a dozen that you can. The challenge comes in finding interesting and involving activities to replace the ones that you've lost. You can be just as joyful and abandoned at chair dancing as you can in traditional dance. Just sit in your chair and let your body and your mind go with the music, keeping time, swaying, moving your feet, your arms, even your shoulders if you wish. It's great. And good exercise, too.

Even my COPD friends in wheel chairs have found compelling things to keep their minds occupied. One of them dabbles in photography, another enjoys cribbage and backgammon, many are actively quilting or in needlepoint groups, one spends time bird watching, another is involved with the community theater. And chair dancing is made to order for wheel chairs.

If you have a window, you can now find bird feeders to fit. Watching cardinals, or the tiny hummingbird is enjoyable.

My own activities (besides working two jobs managing Clambake Celebrations and continuing my marketing consulting practice) include watching movies, meditation and T'ai Chi exercises, bird watching, corresponding with friends and family, volunteer work for our support group, photography, writing, and reading. I adore my needlepoint projects, and keep at least three different canvases going, the more complicated and detailed the pattern, the better. And writing has proved to be a good experience, an especially cathartic one for me. The day is never quite long enough, my interests are wide and varied, and I always run out of energy long before I'm out of something to do.

With friends or family, I'm always up for a game of Scrabble or Monopoly, or Trivial Pursuit or Gin Rummy. At family reunions we've had some splendid poker games, with lots of laughter and good-natured bantering. My grandsons are eager to show up at Gram's house with their newest board game, which they enjoy teaching me. And my daughter has given me a number of grown-up coloring books, beautifully detailed pictures of sea life or Tolkien's Hobbit to be colored in with colored pencils or (my personal favorite) felt-tip pens in brilliant shades. A wonderful activity for a rainy afternoon or a lazy Sunday morning.

Admittedly, these activities are more sedentary than I used to do. But, so what? The only physical activities that I really miss are walking and swimming.

One thing I have learned since becoming ill, it is a waste of time grieving for activities that are no longer possible. There must be at least 10,000 more things to do. I am grateful that my life has been so full, and that I have been able to travel the world and to exercise my options. Maybe some of those beloved activities have been taken away in order for me to have 10,000 other choices.

Traveling

Planning to Travel

Travel with advanced COPD, even with mild COPD, takes some planning. How much extra planning you will have to do depends on the way you want to travel. You rarely see someone on supplemental oxygen traveling on public conveyances. I believe that the main reason is not knowing how to set up and accomplish a trip successfully.

1 Make your plans known to your doctor and request advice. Be sure that your doctor agrees you are well enough to travel.

2 Make sure that you have more than enough medications for the entire trip.

3 Allow for frequent rest periods and emergencies.

Don't be intimidated by the potential hazards of travel. Just take steps to avoid problems. But don't avoid the trip. The golden rule is to book your reservations by telephone and follow up every detail in writing, preferably by fax. And insist on written or faxed confirmations.

While it may be a hassle to have to go to such lengths, it is all worth the effort when your trip goes well.

Since having been diagnosed with lung disease, I have made many trips, both long and short, for business and for pleasure. Traveling with oxygen equipment presents a special set of challenges. Each time I have boarded a plane or train, or checked into a hotel, I have learned something. This cumulative experience may be helpful to you in planning your next trip.

Deciding on a Destination Oxygen Supplier

If you have been prescribed oxygen, arrange oxygen and equipment in your destination city. Professional help is available if you don't want to make all the arrangements yourself. National Oxygen Travel Service (NOTS) in Dayton, Ohio provides oxygen and medical equipment travel services nationally and internationally. They are established specifically to help travelers with their oxygen arrangements. To use their services, your local home/health care oxygen provider needs to become a member of NOTS. A yearly fee must be paid by your oxygen provider, then a fee of $35 must be paid by you for each round-trip that NOTS arranges. This fee is usually offset by the favorable rates NOTS negotiates for liquid oxygen at your destination.

Billing is handled by your local oxygen provider, which means that your insurance will cover your oxygen needs during your trip, except on airplanes, where you pay directly to the airlines.

Booking a trip becomes as simple as requesting a NOTS Passport Planner from your member health/care provider, and faxing the information to NOTS offices in Dayton.

Making Your Own Arrangements

To make arrangements on your own, learn about your destination. Find the names and numbers of companies that provide oxygen and who rent the equipment you need for a short period. Your oxygen provider at home should be able to provide you with suppliers at your destination, or check websites for oxygen suppliers. Also get the name of a person at the company you select.

Phone several oxygen companies at your destination for important facts:

• Can they provide liquid oxygen?

- Do they accept your insurance coverage?
- Is their brand of oxygen equipment compatible with yours?
- Will you be comfortable filling the portable and setting up the equipment?

Informing the supplier

Whether you are making your own arrangements or using NOTS:

- Write or type concise, well-organized details of your trip, then fax it to your contact.
- Give your requirements:
  Your liter flow usage
  Whether you use nasal cannula or face mask
  Type of nasal cannula you prefer
  How much plastic tubing you'll require
  Whether you need a humidifier bottle attachment for sterilized water.
- Request confirmation of all arrangements by return fax.
- Make a list of the days and times of your arrivals and departures, where you'll be staying, and where you'd like the stationary tank set up. Give the list to your home/health care provider or fax to the supplier at your destination.
- Provide a copy of your prescription for oxygen, your doctor's name and phone number, and the name of your regular oxygen provider.

Confirming delivery

Make a file folder for each trip and keep all reservation confirmations, tickets, charge slips and return faxes for a trip in a single folder. Take the folder with you on your trip. You'll need telephone numbers and names if anything goes wrong. Make several photocopies of your prescription for oxygen and keep them in the file.

The trip files also serve as tax records.

Confirming delivery with your hosts

If you are planning to stay with friends or family, let them know about the arrangements for delivery of oxygen and equipment. Check their addresses and phone numbers before giving them to the supplier. For a hotel, make the same arrangements, but include the hotel concierge or head of security in your plans, and use either the concierge or someone who will be on duty from the security department as your contact for the oxygen company.

Reliability

On a trip to Dallas to attend a conference and visit with my family I arranged to stay at my sister Sonja's home. Everything was confirmed with the oxygen company in writing, by fax, a week before the trip, and Sonja was familiar with the oxygen drill. I had used the Dallas company before, and instructed them to set up the stationary equipment at Sonja's house before my arrival, and to fill a portable stroller unit for Sonja to bring to me at the airport. Sonja just needed reminding about how to fill the portable.

On my return to Cape Cod, I was met by the same driver who had brought me to the airport. This time, he stopped by my office to pick up a filled portable unit from my daughter.

I know that these arrangements sound daunting, but the end results were entirely worth it. I enjoyed the buzz and activity as a conference attendee, and loved the opportunity to visit with my friends and family. A well planned trip can be a truly wonderful experience. Just plan all the logistics, get them in writing from everyone involved, and you'll be fine.

Your own research should include getting specific information for disabled travelers. Air Carrier Access rules provide for equal or comparable accommodation for all passengers. But air travelers also have responsibilities, such as providing notice of special needs. Airline and consumer rights and responsibilities are outlined in the brochure, *New Horizons for the Air Traveler with a Disability*. Accommodations and facilities at more than 500 airports worldwide are listed in the brochure, *Access Travel: Airports*. To order these brochures, send your name, address and the title of the brochure to: Consumer Information Center, Pueblo, Colorado 81009.

Emergencies

Beyond arranging oxygen, plan for contingencies. Several members of our support group have made trips to Florida for the winter. They report that the single biggest problem is finding a pulmonologist who will agree to see them when they run into trouble during their stay. Several of them have come down with viruses or other infections, even in the warmth of Florida.

Before you travel, ask your pulmonologist or primary care doctor to refer you to a specialist at your destination. Then as soon as you've settled in call that doctor's office and arrange to be seen before an emergency occurs. That way, if the unforeseen happens, the specialist knows you and can have you admitted to hospital under their care.

Oxygen for Air Travel

As all jet airliner cabins are pressurized, and as the cabins in smaller aircraft are not, the oxygen available in any airliner cabin is less than at sea level. Airliner cabins are not pressurized to sea level, but to a much higher altitude.

Many people think that you can just use the oxygen masks above the seat on an airplane, if you need extra oxygen during flight, but this is not the case. The airline must provide you with a separate cylinder of oxygen exclusively for your use, and they can vary the liter flow as either Low flow (two liters per minute), or High flow (four liters per minute).

Passengers are not allowed to take their own portable oxygen units on board. However most airlines are very accommodating in arranging supplemental oxygen, but some are better than others.

The airlines require about two weeks notice to guarantee oxygen arrangements. So this pretty much negates spur-of-the-moment trips. All airline companies have departments that handle special medical needs. After your first trip with an airline, it will probably maintain your information and medical requirements in a database that can be called up when you travel with them again. But whether you need to start from scratch, or check the records each time you plan to fly, be sure that all details are current and correct.

The Medical Assistance people from the airline will contact you within a week of your trip to get information. By this time, you should have your ticket, with the flight numbers, times of arrival and departure, and destinations. The airline also needs a copy of your prescription for oxygen, and many of them request a letter from your doctor stating that you are well enough to travel.

Airlines charge for the oxygen they provide in-flight. You are charged by flight segment, so if you are traveling to Los Angeles from Boston, with a stop-over in Chicago or Dallas you will have to pay for two segments each way. If you fly non-stop, and one canister of oxygen is enough, you are charged for one flight segment. The usual charge is $75 per segment. The oxygen for a trip to Los Angeles with a stop-over or plane change costs $150 each way, non-stop is $75 each way.

The charges for inflight oxygen can be paid by credit card or personal check, but the airlines will not accept reimbursement by insurance carriers. When you check in at the ticket counter of your departure airport, pay for *all* of your oxygen segments, so that you don't have to pay at each check-in. Your receipt will show that all segments have been paid, and the amount paid in case you can get reimbursed. Some insurance companies cover such expenses, some do not.

Between Flights

For those on supplemental oxygen 24 hours a day, the problem of oxygen to and from the airport, and at your destination airport is a tough one. It is possible to crate and ship an empty portable, but this won't do any good on arrival, because there is no way to uncrate and fill it at the airport.

The airlines are not responsible for providing oxygen on the ground, so if you have a layover, be prepared to go without oxygen until you board the plane again. If you have to change planes, it is a good idea to request in advance, or upon check-in at the departure airport, a wheelchair with an attendant to help you get to the next departure gate. Do this even if you are not wheel-chair dependent, as a rush through a busy airport is not healthy for anyone with lung disease. Don't be shy, it can save a lot of unnecessary wear and tear. But, do plan ahead to avoid long, frustrating waits at the gate when you have a close connection.

When I had a tight connection in Chicago, and was concerned about getting to the connecting gate without oxygen, and in a hurry, I was met by a supervisor from American Airlines Special Services department, and escorted to the next gate in one of those zippy little carts. Imagine the scene if I had not arranged in advance to be met. I would have had to rush to the next gate, without supplemental oxygen, and carrying my carry-on luggage. That would have been an invitation for trouble.

Airline Seating

Seat selection is important. Aisle seats are best for people with COPD. You will not be allowed seating at the bulkhead because there is no place for the oxygen tank (an E-cylinder fitted into a case), or by emergency exits for safety reasons. Avoid middle seats. The airline's oxygen tank is placed underneath the seat in front of you, and in the middle seat you are jammed in. The window seat is difficult to get out of when you have to go to the lavatory.

Flight attendants are very helpful, particularly when treated with courtesy and respect. If you have ordered a special meal, let a flight attendant know as soon as you are settled in your seat, so they know where to bring it when food service begins.

I have flown more than a million miles on American Airlines, many of those since my diagnosis. Given the choice, first class is best for maximum comfort, if you can afford it. There is ample room for you and your oxygen, and you'll get much more care and attention from the flight attendants. If you are traveling by plane only once a year or so, you may prefer to go first class. I get most of my upgrades to first class through my frequent flyer membership.

To and From the Airport

Because I travel alone, I usually have a driver booked to drive me from Cape Cod to either the Boston or Providence airport for departure. The driver must accompany me all the way to the gate and stay with me until I board the plane and am hooked up to the airline's oxygen tank. At that point, my driver leaves, taking my portable oxygen tank with him. I make arrangements for someone to meet me at the destination airport with a filled portable unit. Usually, it is the company I've contracted for my oxygen needs during my stay. This can be expensive. I have been charged as much as $150 just to have someone meet me at the arrival gate with a portable unit. The usual charge is more like $45. But it depends entirely on the company. Even firms that are part of a nationwide chain like Apria Health Care Systems vary their charges for meeting airline passengers. And unfortunately, not all of them are entirely reliable about such a commitment, either.

Small unpressurized planes are not recommended for people with COPD. They do not provide supplemental oxygen on these flights, and their unpressurized cabins can be dangerous for severely-impaired diffusion capabilities. You could lose consciousness during the flight.

Oxygen for Car Travel

Car trips can be a lot of fun, especially if you plan your trip as a wandering adventure. Use automobile forays to get out during the season changes, check out the turning leaves throughout New England in the fall, or visit the Grand Canyon in the spring, before heat and hordes of other vacationers become factors. And no matter where you are in North America, there are winding back roads that will lead you to pastoral scenes, simple pleasures and delightful people. Remember to take along your camera.

If you visit the Grand Canyon or any altitude above 2500 feet, check with your doctor ahead of time. You are likely to need oxygen for the time you are there, or you may need to increase your usual flow rate.

Car trips are easy because you can pace yourself according to how you are feeling. Unlike traveling by air or by train, if you need to stop and rest for awhile, you can. And if you spot an interesting place, you can just pull off, bring out your picnic basket and enjoy the rest.

One year my sister and I planned a trip in the fall, by car to Maine. We planned to do our Christmas shopping at some outlet malls. This was an easy trip to plan, and actually went off without a hitch. First I sent away for information from the Maine Tourist Board, and received a thick catalog of places to stay, and to shop. Then I booked reservations at places to stay after carefully plotting our course on a detailed map. Our itinerary included stops and accommodations for a week's trip.

Next, I called my oxygen provider and explained about my planned trip to Maine. They outfitted me with a small stationary tank filled with liquid oxygen that fit into the back of my Jeep Cherokee, and secured it with bungee cords. I posted an Oxygen In Use sign in the back window of my car. The only danger in driving a car with an oxygen tank in it is being hit from behind. The tank could explode, especially in a fire.

We ran plastic tubing from the back of the Jeep across the back seat, and over the headrest into the front, and then I put the nasal cannula on. I prefer driving to being a passenger, and it was really no different than driving around the Cape with my small portable unit beside me.

The small stationary tank only held enough oxygen for about three days at two liters per minute. So I made arrangements with an oxygen-supply company in Bangor to come to our hotel for a refill after three days. We had a wonderful time.

Oxygen for Train or Bus Travel

I highly recommend travel by train if you have COPD. Once you are comfortably seated, this kind of trip is relaxing, lots of fun and adventure, and very easy. Most of my experience has been up and down the east coast on AMTRAK, and each trip has been a pleasure. Little can go wrong with train travel; the accommodations are comfortable, spacious, and even include sleeper reservations for long trips.

You can bring along your own oxygen in portable tanks. AMTRAK asks that you bring along enough for your trip, plus a little extra in case of delays. With reserved oxygen waiting for you at your hotel, your portable oxygen stroller that you've traveled with on the train should get you there with a bit to spare, if you've calculated correctly, and if you are on time. Let AMTRAK know that you'll be traveling with oxygen when you make your reservations, although I've forgotten to do that when booking, and no one has ever said anything about it on the train.

You can use an oxygen saver with your portable tank, to nearly double oxygen time.

I can drive to the train station in Providence, Rhode Island, from Cape Cod, about one and a half hours, take the train from Providence to Manhattan's Penn Station, about three and a half hours on the Express, take a taxi to my midtown hotel, and arrive with a cushion of about 45 minutes in my portable. Piece of cake!

Having learned that I can come and go from New York City has been a blessing. I accept consulting accounts in the city that require my personal appearance from time to time. And I enjoy, once again, the marvelous bounty that New York has to offer in the way of theater, museums, restaurants and shopping, and many friends.

Train vs Plane

Before discovering the ease of train travel, I attempted several trips to New York by air. Flights from Cape Cod to New York were only available on small, non-jet, non-pressurized planes, which meant I had to travel without supplemental oxygen. I found this nerve-wracking and traumatic, and always landed at my destination with a killer headache.

Train travel is somewhat liberating for me, opening up possibilities that I thought were gone forever. And you can travel alone, without a companion, if your health is good enough. Conductors and other AMTRAK personnel are really dependable about helping with luggage and oxygen units. When you check in at the ticket counter, you can request a red-cap to help at your destination station, and help will be waiting when you disembark.

Bus

Traveling by bus, theoretically, should be a close second to train travel, because you are allowed to bring aboard your own oxygen unit.

This is one method of travel that I cannot personally report on extensively, since I have only taken one day trip by bus. It was fairly comfortable, leaving the driving to someone else, but I was bothered by fumes from the bus exhaust.   *JVT*

Hotels

To successfully book your stay at a hotel, get the name of a person in Special Arrangements, Hotel Security or the name of a Concierge. Make all of your special arrangements through that person after you've made your reservation. Let that person know that you'll be giving their name to the oxygen provider as the contact for setting up your oxygen equipment before your arrival. If you find the arrangements satisfactory on arrival, tip the contact person, then tip again on departure. They'll remember you.

Only experience will help you select hotels with superior concierge and security service, and those with handicap accessible entrances and no stairs. So it is smart to keep a file on the hotels that you've stayed in, in each of the cities you visit. Just place a copy of the hotel's brochure in your folder, and make notes on it for your next booking.

You may find it worthwhile to join a membership program of a large hotel chain with many different locations, such as Sheraton's Gold International Club. The charge is about $25 for a year, and membership entitles you to suite upgrades and to many other services, including attentive floor concierges who are eager to help. Most of the large chains offer some version of a frequent-guest program.

Planning Vacations

Don't be shy about planning vacations that require air travel, or train travel, or any other method of transport. There are always ways to make it work, so choose a vacation that will provide you with the escape that you need. Be sure that all of your written arrangements have been clearly understood and accepted in writing. Then, *go for it!*

None of us should be deprived of the pleasures of occasional travel, just because we have obstructive airway disease. We are not contagious. We are capable of finding our own solutions for any problems that may face us during a vacation. We need the socialization of friends and family, and like anyone else, we respond well to the anticipation of seeing new sights and old friends. Indulge yourself in a vacation trip at least once a year. It will help to recharge your batteries to come back and face the daily grind of living with a chronic illness. Stay within your budget, of course, but give yourself something to look forward to. You'll find that all of the planning to make a trip is well worth it.

Cruises

Cruises are my first choice for a vacation because of the wide range of trips, accommodations, ports of call, comfort, social activities, and general accessibility. And because it is relatively easy to arrange for oxygen and equipment, cruises are relaxing, leisurely, pampering and romantic, even if you are traveling alone. And they are all-inclusive. Almost all arrangements are made ahead of time, so you can just relax.

Cruises are also wonderful because your room is close by to take short rests during the day, if you need to. And there is nothing better than ocean air for impaired lungs. Cruise directors are always glad to help you set up a special diet, and the ships all have terrific gyms and exercise equipment. Many of them have full-fledged spa facilities, including spa-approved cuisine. There are both indoor and outdoor pools, and most cruise lines include regular pool exercise classes.

If you don't wish to interrupt your day in the sun by taking a snooze in your cabin, there is always a comfortable deck chair. You can catch up on your reading while you rest and enjoy the fresh, moist air. You needn't worry about bringing a load of books along, there are lots of good choices in the ship's library.

Entertainment on cruise ships is legendary. There are marvelous shows, movies and live performances to choose from in the evening. Every piano and library bar offers live entertainment: musicians, comedians, dancers, lecturers, etc. You can choose amongst bingo games, casinos, dance lessons, costume parties, bridge and backgammon games, or take leisurely strolls around the ship in the early mornings, and the aerobics classes in the heated indoor pool. There are midnight buffets, afternoon high teas, brunches, and all the regular meals.

You can be as busy or as quiet as you choose. You can simply let it be known that you prefer to stay by yourself, if that is your choice. Everyone understands the need for private time, even on vacation.

Alone vs. groups

Traveling alone on a cruise can be lovely, if you just wish to get away from it all, to spend your time with spur-of-the-moment activities or napping in your cabin. You don't have to check in with anyone, and if you feel like skipping a meal or a cocktail gathering, just do it.

After all of my years of travel, I am convinced that the fewer people in any travel party, the simpler the trip.

Traveling alone is easiest, because you can do whatever you wish without having to consider another person. Large travel groups, like tour groups, are the worst, because they have to be conducted on schedule. Flexibility is non-existent on a tour group, except for those days that are purposely set aside as free time.

But cruises are romantic environments, so traveling alone may not be for you. There are always fewer single men than women, so it is not ideal if you are a single woman seeking male companionship, but for single men, it may be just the thing.

However, traveling alone on a cruise is certainly not a sentence of solitude. You are sure to meet many nice people from all over the world, many with the same interests.

I've met people on cruises that I've stayed in touch with, enjoying our correspondence very much.

While I've loved the cruises I've been on in the Caribbean, Greek Islands, the coast of Mexico, and the Mediterranean, the best ship I have sailed on was the QE2, in all her majesty and grace, and with just the right size passenger list to provide the finest service and food. On some larger ships there are problems of having to stand in line for table seating at meals, for tickets for port excursions, and for other activities.

Resorts

Another relaxing vacation is to book a stay at a resort. It really doesn't matter where—ocean, mountains, desert—as much as what you want when you get there. If you are looking for quiet with wonderful food and warm hospitality, you can select from thousands of inns and bed-and-breakfasts, all over North America and much of the rest of the world.

If your idea of a terrific vacation is an elegant resort with all the amenities, you can certainly be accommodated. The important thing is to plan, and to provide your requirements to the management of your destination in plenty of time.

Spas

Even with restrictions on your physical activities, you can enjoy a fabulous week at a fitness resort or health spa.

For more than 10 years, I booked a week each year at The Golden Door in Escondido, California. I always returned feeling healthier, rested, more fit, certainly more peaceful and serene.

Spas and fitness centers understand completely about having to customize for each person, particularly those with debilitating illnesses. These facilities are great places for learning Yoga and meditation, and they provide soothing body massages with herbal wraps, facials, and healing Jacuzzi baths. Your exercise program is fitted to your abilities and restrictions. Although guests with breathing problems cannot be put into aerobic dance classes, they can function very well in many other activities, including pool exercise. They probably cannot play tennis, but can go on walks with no inclines.

You can visit a health spa alone, or with friends. If you go alone, you'll meet new friends quickly and have all the company you want during your stay. Friendships blossom, and you're sure to come away with new chums and contacts. You'll probably meet some of the same people at the resort, same time next year.

The best thing about a stay at a spa is that the packing could not be simpler. For example, the Golden Door provides warm-ups, kimonos, exercise wear such as shorts and T-shirts. All you need to bring is your tennis shoes, nightie, bathing suit, and a couple of pairs of slacks and shirts or sweaters. Even a hair dryer is provided in your room, along with a marvelous sampling of skin care products, shampoos, and lotions. Rooms at The Golden Door are Japanese-style garden suites, with a private meditation garden or pond for each guest. The bathrooms are equipped with oversized, fluffy bath sheets for bathing and to cover a lounge chair by the pool. Breakfast is brought to your room as soon as you return from your early morning walk. Other meals may be taken with the other guests in the dining room, or privately in your own room, if you prefer.

The staff works with you to plan your nutrition exactly to your requirements. They do all they can to help you lose weight or gain it, as needed. Diet cuisine is simply fabulous, beautifully served and presented. You won't feel deprived, even if you've chosen a 1,500-calorie a day plan. The camaraderie in such a place is remarkable. After a week you'll feel as if you are leaving family behind.

10 Severe Disease and Treatment

Our emphasis on helping COPD people to find the courage to live with the illness has been placed on patient education. More knowledge about this complicated disease will make it easier to live pro-actively, and to avoid, wherever possible, exacerbations. It also makes it less difficult to handle such problems if they do arise. Arm yourself with all the information you can get, in order to be able to take in stride whatever develops.

The following chapter may be painful for you to read and to absorb, because it deals rather graphically with the most serious aspects of lung disease. But it is knowledge that you should have, for your own protection. It is not possible to avoid the realities of COPD by ignoring the possibilities. It is far better to make yourself aware of the risks and the choices. This is also a chapter to share with your spouse or caregivers. They should learn about these issues, so that when choices must be made they will be able to help and support you in your deci-sions.

RC, BN, JVT

Surgical and medical interventions may be helpful in improving failing respira-tion and getting through acute respiratory failure. You should learn about and understand treatment options for severe COPD long before you may need them. You may wish to discuss these options with doctors, a lawyer, and family mem-bers in order to make decisions.

Respiratory Failure

Respiratory failure occurs when the lungs are no longer able to keep normal oxy-gen levels in the blood and get rid of carbon dioxide. Diagnosis of respiratory failure is usually made when lung disease has become severe.

Acute respiratory failure occurs when some new process starts, which further damages the lungs either temporarily or permanently.

Chronic respiratory failure is the result of a steady downhill course of lung disease and often occurs without acute illness.

Acute Respiratory Failure

Acute respiratory failure usually occurs over a period of hours or days. Diagnosis is based on distress and abnormal arterial blood gases. The person is always short of breath, and usually has to sit up to breathe, as lying down increases a feeling of smothering. The person is often confused and may not know where they are or the date. At times, the fingernails may be bluish due to lack of oxygen. There may be gurgling, wheezing or other audible sounds with breathing.

Blood gases show a low oxygen level. It may be difficult to bring the level up to an acceptable value just by giving extra oxygen. Often the person needs to be observed in the intensive care unit (ICU) and may need breathing support with a mechanical ventilator.

The most frequent cause of respiratory failure is exacerbation of COPD, with either an increase in bronchospasm recognized by wheezing, or by acute bronchitis with increased inflammation of the bronchial tubes, with or without infection. Another common cause of exacerbations is pneumonia, caused by bacterial infection, viral infection such as influenza, or other causes.

Not as common, but potentially catastrophic, is lung collapse or *pneumothorax*. This occurs with COPD mainly because some parts of the lungs are so thinned by emphysema that one of these thin areas bursts. When this occurs, air leaks out of the hole in the lung, collecting outside the lung and inside the chest wall. This air exerts back pressure on the thin lung and causes it to collapse. Usually when this happens, the person has sudden pleurisy or severe chest pain when inhaling or coughing, and quickly becomes short of breath.

Heart disease may also cause respiratory failure. If the heart is not pumping effectively, this may result in extra fluid backing up in the lung. With already-damaged lungs, this fluid may be enough to cause the lungs to fail. Giving too much fluid after surgery, in case of excessive bleeding from the intestinal tract, or when treating some other disease may cause the same sort of problem.

Chronic Respiratory Failure

Chronic respiratory failure is usually not associated with an acute change. Usually the person is going gradually downhill, having more and more trouble with normal activity. Diagnosis of respiratory failure is based on blood gases which show low oxygen, but in contrast to the acute situation, it is usually easy to get the level up to normal with a little extra oxygen. Also, blood gases generally reveal an elevation of carbon dioxide, showing that the lungs are failing to keep up with excreting the body's main waste product.

Chronic respiratory failure rarely reverses. However, people can live for years with respiratory failure, particularly using continuous oxygen therapy and managing lung dysfunction by learning all that they can about their disease and its treatment, and by *practising what they learn. Just learning is not enough. Consistent practice is essential, and so is being very consistent with interventions.*

Treatment of Respiratory Failure

Treatment of respiratory failure has three parts:

- Treating the lung disease
- Treating the cause of acute respiratory failure
- Supporting the person through recovery.

Lung disease is treated with the same medications discussed in *Medications for COPD* on page 69, including:

- Bronchodilators to open the air tubes
- Steroids to reduce inflammation and further open the air tubes
- Medications to liquefy lung mucus so it may be cleared.

The cause of acute respiratory failure is treated with whatever is appropriate: antibiotics, a chest tube, or diuretic therapy.

Treatment Options

Life support: Support may require very aggressive therapy such as placing a tube in the windpipe and then completely controlling *ventilation* or breathing with a machine called a *respirator*.

Respiratory support: Another choice is the use of a bi-level positive airway pressure device with a tight-fitting face mask to deliver air under pressure which pushes the breath in so the person does not need to work as hard to breathe. This is becoming a common way to support a person for several hours or a few days, giving medicines time to work. See *Respiratory support with a non-invasive ventilator* on page 190.

Chest tube for pneumothorax: Pneumothorax may require treatment by chest tube. A tube is inserted between the ribs, inside the chest cavity but outside the lungs. Suction is used to evacuate the free air and pull on the lung to expand it. This tube may have to stay in the chest a long time, since the lung is so thinned it is hard for it to heal.

Figure 39   Using a chest tube to expand a collapsed lung

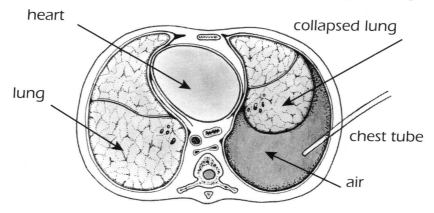

A tube may be inserted into the chest to remove trapped air and thus allow a collapsed lung to expand.

Sometimes feeding must be done with a tube through the nose into the stomach. Sometimes the person can eat. Medications to support blood pressure and control heart rhythm may be required. Discuss these options with your doctor at your routine checkups. It is important for you to have a clear understanding of what your doctor is trying to accomplish and the options available.

Surgical Options

Lung Transplant

Until recently, there was little to offer people with severe COPD when medicines no longer were effective in easing difficult breathing. In the past 10-15 years, however, two different types of surgery have become available. Neither is a cure for COPD, nor can the surgery be performed on everyone.

The newest procedure is lung-reduction surgery. This type of operation has been performed only since 1994 and there are still many questions about how well it works and how long the good effects last. In carefully selected people it results in greatly improved ability to breathe and increased ability to be active.

Lung transplant is also a procedure useful only in carefully selected people who have the type of disease which will respond to transplant without too great a risk of infection, and who have no other diseases which would complicate the transplant. This procedure is very stressful psychologically since it requires a strict medical regimen over several years. It is not for everyone.

Lung Volume Reduction Surgery

Although lung transplant surgery has been available for several years, it became clear early on that only a few of the people with severe COPD would be eligible, and even in those who underwent the procedure, survival was often limited. Because of these problems, attempts are being made to find a simpler and more successful surgical treatment.

Emphysema causes enlargement of the alveoli, the tiny balloons at the end of the bronchial tubes. When these alveoli enlarge, they do not push and pull the air in and out as they should, and the elastic tissue which forms the walls of the alveoli is destroyed, so that it no longer pulls on the bronchial tubes to keep them open. These changes are more completely explained in the chapter on *Breathing and COPD*.

Almost since emphysema was recognized as a disease, surgeons have been trying to find ways to cure it. They have not succeeded. But surgical treatment may be an option in some cases. With severe emphysema, the lung can't stretch to breathe in air, but if the badly damaged parts of the lung can be removed by surgery, several things happen:

- The lung is smaller, fits into the space between the ribs better, and can stretch out as air is breathed in. Very little space is available for breathing in the lung with emphysema, see *Lung volume in healthy and emphysemic lungs* on page 36, surgery creates more space for breathing.
- With a smaller lung, the diaphragm can work more efficiently and effectively to move air in and out. The other muscles around the ribs and the neck may not have to do as much work. This can help shortness of breath, especially after arm activity.

- Removal of alveoli so stretched that they do not work means you have to do less work to breathe. Before surgery, effort was wasted and didn't bring oxygen to the body. After surgery, the work of breathing goes to better parts of the lung, so it is more efficient.
- When you cut out the really damaged parts of the lung and the little bronchial tubes which are in these areas, you leave good lung with wider bronchial tubes. You can breathe through a hose again, instead of a straw.

This surgery has been performed many times. Most people who have the surgery are less short of breath and able to be more active. Often they no longer require regular oxygen, and need to use oxygen only when they exercise or not at all. Recent studies[1] are demonstrating that this surgery reduces the height of

Figure 40   Before and after lung volume reduction surgery

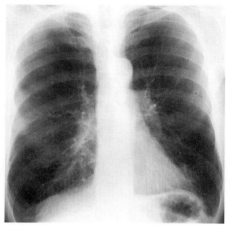

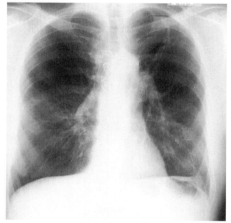

This frontal chest radiograph (x-ray) of a 70 year old man with emphysema shows an enlarged lung and chest, and a flattened diaphragm. Radiographs courtesy Julie E. Takasugi, M.D.

After surgery, the radiograph of the same man shows changes including: overall reduction in lung height and reduction of the diameter of the chest. In many cases, the diaphragm shows an improved arc.

the lung, reduces the diameter of the chest, allows the diaphragm to become more normal with a greater rounding or arc, and results in an improvement in symptoms and respiratory function tests. The respiratory muscles are no longer over-stretched and thus may be able to work better.

Candidates for surgery

However:

Only one out of every three or four people can have the surgery. It works in people with emphysema, not those with mostly bronchitis or asthma.

- Often the surgery cannot be performed in people who have had pneumonia or other infections, or lung surgery.
- Like any other surgery, it is riskier when you are sicker or when you have other diseases.

1. Personal communication from Julie E. Takasugi, MD, Department of Radiology, Puget Sound Health Care System, Seattle, WA; Takasugi et al, "Lung-Volume Reduction Surgery for Diffuse Emphysema: Radiologic Assessment of Changes in Thoracic Dimensions," *Journal of Thoracic Imaging,* 13:36-41, 1998

- Most surgeons will not even consider this surgery if you have not stopped smoking for at least six months. A most important consideration is whether or not you continue to be exposed to cigarette smoke.
- Your lung specialist must work with your surgeon to decide if you are a good candidate for the operation and when to do the surgery.

Since surgery is not always successful and is not without risks, the decision to try surgery is usually based on shortness of breath severe enough to really interfere with daily life. This means you can't even do normal daily activities like light housework, carrying groceries, or walking slowly on the level.

Another very important factor is your overall physical condition and muscle strength. Active participation in a physical therapy and rehabilitation program before and after surgery is usually required. This may be carried out at the hospital, at a therapy center, or at home, but it seems to make a big difference in an person's ability to regain strength and mobility.

Breathing tests like spirometry are administered, x-rays, CAT scans or other pictures of the lungs are obtained, and your ability to exercise is tested in the laboratory. These tests must show that the major reason you are short of breath is emphysema, and not any other type of lung or heart disease.

Risks

You may have the surgery and not be better afterward. You may even be worse. Even if the operation is successful, you may have to stay in the hospital for a while with tubes into your chest between your ribs. And there is a four to seven percent chance that you may die as a result of the procedure.

Choices

There are very different ways to do the surgery. The choice depends on the surgeon's preference and experience, the type of disease you have, whether there is a problem of another type (such as previous infection) in only one lung, and your overall medical condition. One procedure is done like open heart bypass surgery, where the incision is down the center front of the chest. Both lungs are operated on at once. Another way to do the surgery is on one lung at a time, either by putting a tube between the ribs through a small incision, or by operating through an incision directly into the cavity around the lung, and removing damaged lung tissue with a laser or a stapler.

The effects of surgery may last only a few years before the disease gets as bad as it was before surgery. The National Institutes of Health are carrying out a nationwide study in many different medical centers of the United States to find out how good the surgery is and how long it lasts.

This surgical procedure is still considered experimental by Medicare, and thus not covered by most insurance carriers.

Lung Transplant

Another option is lung transplant. If this procedure is successful, it offers a chance at a normal life with minimal limitations. Unfortunately, this is not nearly as successful a procedure as is kidney or heart transplant. While four out of five people survive for one year after lung transplant, survival for five years is often less than one out of two. Of the people who live, many have persistent breathing problems.

Many insurance policies do not cover lung transplant. Transplant is very expensive, with most institutions demanding $400,000 before hospital admission.

Candidates

Transplant is usually refused for people over 55-60 years old, as the procedure and recovery are so strenuous. Since most transplants are done with a single lung and the donor's other organs are transplanted to other people, people with heart disease who may also need heart transplant are refused transplant. People on large doses of steroids, or those with a history of many respiratory infections may also be refused due to the high risk of complications. Transplant is most often used for the young, otherwise healthy person with alpha1-antitrypsin disease.

Follow-up

Following the transplant, you have to religiously follow a strict schedule of medications, breathing tests, x-rays and check-ups. Medications are aimed at preventing the body from reacting to the transplanted lung or rejecting it. These medications cause the body's defenses, the immune system, to be less active. As a result, the chances of infection are greatly increased. Many transplant programs require the recipient to undergo bronchoscopy, a direct look at the inside of the bronchial tubes through a fiber-optic instrument, at scheduled intervals, and for any fever or sign of infection or rejection of the new lung.

Survival after lung transplants is improving as experience increases in handling medications to prevent rejection. Knowledge of the types of infections likely to occur and the best methods to diagnose and treat these infections is much more exact than in the past. We hope that lung transplant will be easier to tolerate and more successful in the years ahead.

Ventilation Assistance

If lung reduction surgery for emphysema, described earlier, is not an option and your lung disease is very severe and worsening, then what is left? One possibility is the use of a machine to help do the breathing for you, that is, a mechanical support device to help make breathing easier for some or all of the time. These devices are most frequently used to tide a person over a short but severe episode of illness, where the situation is expected to get better. They may also be used permanently, where the situation is not expected to improve. The human, social, and financial costs of long-term respiratory support are high. There must be a very supportive home or long term care environment with knowledgeable caretakers. The financial burden is substantial and not completely covered by insurance.

Using Positive Air Pressure and Mask

The easiest mechanical device to use delivers positive pressure through a mask over either the nose, or the nose and mouth. This is called a bi-level positive airway pressure device. Positive pressure blows air into the lungs with little effort. Sometimes exhaling is also assisted by positive pressure to keep the bronchial tubes from collapsing. In COPD, these devices are used most often to allow someone who is worn out by infection or other exacerbations to rest.

Figure 41   Respiratory support with a non-invasive ventilator

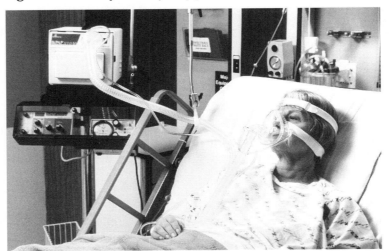

A BiPAP® made by Respironics (bi-level positive airway pressure) device delivers air through a full-face mask to assist breathing.

A nasal or full-face mask may be worn for several hours at a time, or continuously. A mask is occasionally used at night to allow recovery from the fatigue of extra effort to breathe with severe COPD during the day. These devices, pictured in Figure 41, have many drawbacks. Talking, eating, and coughing are very difficult if not impossible while wearing them. They are uncomfortable due to the tight fit and can cause skin breaks and sores. Pressure in the mask may cause air to leak out and irritate the eyes. Adjusting the pressure may be very difficult, requiring a great deal of trial and error. If the pressure is not correctly adjusted, the mask may even make shortness of breath worse, leading to a feeling of suffocation.

On the other hand, people who become used to wearing a mask find they can relax and rest, making the time off the mask much more comfortable.

The mask is impractical for someone unconscious or uncooperative or who has a large volume of sputum. In these circumstances, a breathing machine such as a respirator or mechanical ventilator is used to totally take over breathing responsibility until you can breathe on your own.

Using a Tube in the Windpipe

A respirator or mechanical ventilator provides life support to people who have a high likelihood of dying without the use of the machine. If successfully used, the machine does the work of the lungs for days, weeks, months or even years. Experience with these machines is widespread and they are valuable for supporting people with COPD. In using such life support, the hope is that given treatment and time, the person will return to the functional level they had.

Using a breathing machine for life support is no guarantee of survival. Many complications can result from life support, and sometimes disease is so severe that medications and machines do not help.

An example of a situation where life support might be used is for a person with stable emphysema, who can function well enough to be at home, getting along with the aid of family members, although exercise is limited. Should that person develop pneumonia, the insult from the pneumonia may be enough to cause

Figure 42   Respirator to provide life support

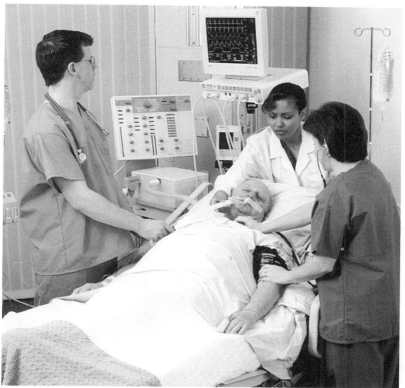

A respirator or mechanical ventilator provides life support to people who have a high likelihood of dying without the use of the machine. In using such life support, the hope is that given treatment and time, the person will return to the functional level they had. Respiratory support and patient monitoring equipment shown here is manufactured by Siemens Medical Systems, Inc.

respiratory failure. Using a breathing machine allows the person to rest while the machine does the work of breathing, supporting the person while the pneumonia is treated with antibiotics and other therapy. Gradually the person can assume more and more work to breathe off the mechanical ventilator. This process is called weaning and it allows a gradual resumption of lung work, without tiring by suddenly having to do all the work of breathing. After this, the person will hopefully recover to the medical status before pneumonia. However, emphysema is still there and no less severe than before the pneumonia. The use of mechanical ventilation does not make the basic disease any better.

A disadvantage of vigorous mechanical life support is that the person must be in an intensive care unit (ICU), where the number of visitors and the length of visits are limited. Further, because of the tubes in the windpipe and the need for other measures to provide life support, the person often cannot talk or communicate.

Endotracheal tube

Using mechanical ventilation requires the placement of a large tube, about the size of your little finger, directly into the windpipe or *trachea* through the mouth or the nose and through the vocal cords. With the endotracheal tube in place, it is not possible to make any sounds at all, as no air can come through the vocal cords. Eating with the tube in place is also impossible, as it prevents swallowing. The tube is very uncomfortable, making people feel choked or suffocated. Most awake people will try to pull the tube out, at least at first. Because of efforts to pull the tube out, the person may be heavily sedated, almost unconscious. At times, special medicines may be given to relax the muscles so that no movement is possible.

While the tube is in the windpipe, feeding is by a separate smaller tube inserted through the nose into the stomach or upper small intestine. A liquid diet containing protein, fats and carbohydrates is given through this tube in order to prevent malnutrition and further weakness.

Intravenous or IV lines are needed to give medications. If the veins are not good, a needle must be placed in a vein of the neck or upper chest. A needle may also be placed in an artery in order to accurately measure blood pressure and to show how much oxygen is getting in, and how much carbon dioxide is being removed by ventilation.

Dependence on the ventilator

One fear of mechanical ventilation is that the person never recovers enough to be free of the mechanical ventilator, that is, that the lungs will not be strong enough to take over the work of breathing. The likelihood of this happening is related to disease severity. The less working lung tissue remaining, the lower the chance of successfully removing the ventilator.

The ability to come off the breathing machine may also be determined by the presence of other diseases such as diabetes, heart disease or arthritis which may themselves cause weakness, as well as malnutrition and mental problems such as senility. When there has been a steady downhill progression of lung disease without a sudden change, the likelihood is low of being able to successfully discontinue the breathing machine and restore the person to independent life outside the hospital. In that case, the person may be bound to the machine for the rest of life. The person cannot be weaned from the ventilator.

Many people find this an intolerable situation and do not wish to survive if bound to the ventilator. Others feel differently and wish to live even if the ventilator is required. A person may be disconnected from the ventilator, by their request even though the result of the disconnection may be death.

Tracheostomy

When a ventilator is needed for a prolonged time, a procedure called a *tracheostomy* is often done. This involves placing the breathing tube directly into the windpipe through a hole in the front. This method is similar to transtracheal oxygen delivery, but the catheter tube is much larger and is attached to a respirator (See *Transtracheal oxygen delivery* on page 100). Once this procedure is done, the endotracheal tube can be removed from the mouth or nose, which usually allows the person to eat. Talking is still difficult but can be accomplished through a tube designed for talking or mouthing words to improve communication. If breathing support is no longer needed, the breathing tube can be removed. The opening usually heals closed, leaving a small scar.

Refusing Breathing Assistance

If you do not wish to receive life support with a ventilator, what are the options? This question needs to be addressed directly to your doctor, in order that you, your family, nurses, and other caretakers will all feel that the correct decision has been made. If your lungs have gotten worse, so that breathing is very difficult, you may not wish to remain alive at all costs. Some people have had episodes of life support and do not wish to go through it again. Other diseases may be present and making life uncomfortable.

In years past, we all accepted the idea of dying quietly, hopefully surrounded by loved ones. We accepted this as the natural way for life to end. The fact that artificial support for life is available does not mean that it must be used. Allowing a person to die quietly with minimal interference from medical personnel except to make the person comfortable is often referred to as *death with dignity.*

Accepting Support but Excluding Mechanical Ventilation

In other cases, a person may not wish to be on life support but may wish everything done short of mechanical ventilation. Treat the lung disease vigorously and minimize or withhold sedatives or narcotics which might interfere with recovery. In some cases, because of other medications and even without the use of a breathing machine, a severe bout of disease may get better.

For example, the British almost never put people on breathing machines for life support and most people still survive.

In people with a reasonable hope of recovery, whether or not a breathing machine for life support is used, vigorous treatment of the lung disease is continued. If in spite of treatment severe shortness of breath persists, and the person does not want life support on a breathing machine, then shortness of breath can be treated with narcotics. It is well recognized that morphine and its opiate relatives are the best medications for severe pain, but fewer people are aware that morphine is just as effective in relieving shortness of breath.

Support and the Conservative Approach

If a decision is made to avoid life support, then comfort can be provided with the use of narcotics. No one should have to die with miserable shortness of breath as the alternative to life support. At times, interestingly, because of the inability of the body to get rid of carbon dioxide as the lungs fail, the person may get very sleepy or even go into a coma. Carbon dioxide is a natural sedative and if the person is not uncomfortable with shortness of breath, then narcotics may not be necessary.

An advantage to the conservative approach at the end of life is that families can be with the person for mutual support. A hospice unit in the hospital or special hospice care given in the home may make everyone more accepting of the inevitability of death. Such support can help both the dying person and the family to cope better and to realize that death is a natural event which will come to all of us at some time. Religious support at this time is important for many people and often prevents hopelessness toward the end of life.

Should Breathing be Supported by a Machine?

It is important to stress that there is no right or wrong answer to the question of whether breathing should be supported by a machine. The decision belongs to the person concerned, who usually makes it after discussing it with the doctor and with the support and acquiescence of loved ones (See *Advance Directives: Planning for Difficult Decisions* on page 195).

It is generally accepted in the United States that only if the doctor feels there is no chance of survival of that episode of illness, a *medically hopeless* situation, should the doctor refuse to perform mechanical ventilation if the resources are available. In other countries, different decisions have been made by the society as a whole, such as a policy decision that people with COPD will not generally be ventilated in the event of respiratory failure.

Advance Directives: Planning for Difficult Decisions

Because COPD is a chronic and progressive disease, it may eventually cause death. That is, the lungs can deteriorate so much that the person cannot breathe enough to live. Death is usually preceded by steadily increasing shortness of breath. Instead of difficulty breathing only during exercise or with a cold, shortness of breath is constant, whether you are resting or active. As all therapies become less effective and last a shorter time you are hospitalized more and more frequently.

Life and death decisions should not be rushed, nor should they be made by someone who does not know what you wish. When therapies become less effective, some major decisions need to be made about transplant, life support, and other options. You, your family and the doctor need to thoroughly discuss all these options *before* an emergency, and provide written instructions. Also discuss with the doctor and include in your instructions a circumstance when your brain is functional, but your lungs are not, and you are unable to speak. With COPD, this is the more likely situation.

Your Legal Rights in Health Care

All adult patients in hospitals, skilled nursing facilities, and health care settings have certain rights under the law. In the United States, this includes the right to confidentiality of your personal and medical records and the right to know what treatment you will receive. You also have the right, in the United States, to prepare an *advance directive* stating how you want medical decisions made for you if you lose the ability to make decisions for yourself. There are two types of advance directives:

- Living Will
- Durable Power of Attorney for Health Care.

United States federal law requires hospitals, skilled nursing facilities, hospices, health care agencies, and health maintenance organizations (HMOs) serving people covered by Medicare or Medicaid to give them information about advance directives. They must explain the legal options in making decisions about medical care. However, state laws differ regarding advance directives, so the state health-care organization is required to provide these laws to you and to offer reasonable explanations of the laws.

Similar laws, rights and powers are usual in other English-speaking countries, such as Australia, Canada, England, and Scotland, but may be differently applied and enforced. In non-English-speaking countries, the situation may be quite different. Check with your doctor or a lawyer about your rights.

Living Will

If you reach a point in your life where you cannot make your own decisions, a living will directs health care providers to follow your medical decisions. It is called a living will because it takes effect when you are living. Living will formats vary from state to state so it is important that you request the forms for the state in which you have established your permanent residence.

In other countries such as Canada, a living will may only be used as guidance, not legally enforceable rights and powers. But at least the living will clearly states your wishes.

Durable Power of Attorney for Health Care

In most of the United States, a durable power of attorney for health care is a signed, dated, and witnessed document naming another person to act as your authorized spokesperson for medical decisions. You can include specific statements regarding the care you expect to receive or that you want to avoid. Get the written agreement of the person you choose as your agent to speak for you when you cannot speak for yourself. Discuss your wishes about life support and other issues with your agent so that the written document is clear.

It may be possible to have either two documents or a single, combined document. Check your state or national law.

Is One Better Than the Other?

In the United States the law on honoring an advance directive varies from state to state. However, if you travel, the advance directive will generally be honored in any state. The drawback is that you must make the advance directive known to the medical care provider. If you spend considerable time in two or more states, prepare a set of advance directives for each state and follow each state's requirements concerning the preparation of these documents.

If you travel to another country for significant periods of time, prepare another set of directives according to the laws of that country, and the part of the country in which you stay.

Advance directives can be canceled or changed at any time. Any change or cancellation must be in writing, signed and dated in accordance with the law governing the directive. Give copies of a change to your doctor, lawyer, and other people in a position to be requested to make decisions for you. For example:

- If you have a durable power of attorney, give a copy to the agent or proxy.
- Ask your doctor to make your advance directive part of your permanent medical record. This must include both the office record and the hospital medical record.
- Keep a copy of the advance directive in a safe place where it can be easily and quickly found.
- Keep a copy in your safe deposit box or some other secure area such as the lawyer's office.
- Place a visible small card in your wallet or purse stating that you have an advance directive, where it is located and who your agent or proxy is, if one has been named.

11 Considerations Before Surgery

Factors to Consider before Surgery

People with COPD are usually middle-aged or older, and have often been or still are smokers. These folks may develop the same diseases other people do as they age and may need surgery. But because of abnormalities with breathing which are always present with COPD, any surgery is a problem.

When deciding about surgery other than lung reduction or transplant, consider several factors:

- How bad is the lung function?
- What part of the body is to be operated on and what surgery is to be done?
- What type of anesthesia will be used?
- Is any tissue to be removed?
- How important is the surgery?

Severity of Lung Disease

If the disease is mild, it may not increase the risk of surgery much, if at all. If the disease is severe and the person is not likely to survive long just because of the severity of the lung problems, then surgery is probably not an option.

To decide how bad the lung situation is, lung function is measured. Categorizing lung function as *mildly, moderately* or *severely abnormal* is generally based on the FEV_1 test, the amount of air exhaled in the first second of blowing. The table below shows the relationship between the percent of expected value the person reached and the severity of lung abnormality. The worse the abnormality in lung function, the higher the surgical risk.

Maximal voluntary ventilation is measured by what the person can actually breathe with a major effort. This is determined in the laboratory by how much air can move in and out by really hyperventilating, breathing hard and fast for several seconds, at maximal effort. Some surgeons prefer to have the person

Table 24: Lung function and surgical risk

Lung function	FEV$_1$ as a percent of normal value	Surgical risk
Normal	More than 80%	Not increased
Mild	60 - 80%	Not increased
Moderate	40 - 60%	Somewhat increased
Severe	Less than 40%	Very increased

exercise while they watch. For example, they climb one or more flights of stairs together. This obviously requires the surgeon to be in good shape and very observant.

If lung function measurements indicate that the person has moderate or severe disease, then arterial blood gases are drawn so the lungs' ability to get rid of carbon dioxide can be evaluated. Getting rid of carbon dioxide is a measure not only of lung function but also of the brain's activity in signalling the lung muscles to take a breath. Arterial blood gases are also measured for oxygen in the blood, an important number to guide the anesthesiologist in the operating room.

Surgery and Site

How much risk surgery carries in people with COPD depends on what part of the body is to be operated on and the type and amount of surgery, as well as quality and quantity of lung function.

An operation on the lower leg or neck is unlikely to be very risky, even in someone with severe disease, because the surgery itself will not interfere with the ability of the lungs to breathe, or with coughing. Lung disease does not become worse as a result of such surgery.

A short procedure where an intestinal specialist looks into your swallowing tube and stomach, is not risky.

When a lung specialist looks into your windpipe and bronchial tubes, the risk is usually low, though wheezing and increased shortness of breath may occur.

Operations done high up in the abdomen or in the chest itself, can interfere with the ability to cough and clear out phlegm because of pain causing a reluctance to breathe deeply. For abdomen or chest surgery, the extent of the surgery is very important. *Cholecystectomy*, or gall bladder removal, can be done with an older type of surgery which requires a long incision just below the ribs and pulling the tissue far apart to get to the gall bladder, or gall bladder removal can be performed through four tiny incisions, using fiberoptics to get light into the area and newer techniques to cut out the tissue. This is a surgical technique that can be used on many, but not all people. The risks for these two surgical procedures are not at all the same.

Heart surgery, done by splitting apart the sternum (the hard center cartilage in the front of the chest), is less risky than lung surgery done by making a long incision between the ribs. When you have to get into the chest by cutting between the ribs, this means you have to cut through a lot of nerves and also that the lung will have to collapse as you let air into the chest. The sternum lacks nerves and causes much less pain when it is split. One operation thus causes a lot more pain than the other, difficulty coughing, deep-breathing and clearing out phlegm. However, new anesthesia techniques have cut the risk in this procedure.

Risks with Anesthesia

In general, procedures done under local anesthesia, where the anesthesiologist only deadens the area to be operated on, or with regional anesthesia, where only the nerves leading to the surgical site (usually an arm or leg) are deadened, are not risky for those with lung disease.

Procedures where the person is sedated enough to prevent the procedure from being frightening or painful, but where the person is still awake, also carry a very low risk.

Operations which can be done with low spinal anesthesia, such as some procedures below the waist, carry a low risk as they don't interfere with lung function after the surgery.

Higher risk procedures are those done with spinal anesthesia where the anesthesia has to go above the waist, and those done with general anesthesia. General anesthesia means that you are put completely to sleep, and a tube is placed in your windpipe for breathing. For most of the operation you are in a coma and cannot breathe for yourself so the anesthesiologist has to do it for you. The risk increases because the anesthetic techniques interfere with breathing and with the normal ability of the lungs to clear out mucus. Even a very skilled anesthesiologist cannot clear out phlegm as effectively as you yourself can by deep breathing and coughing. After procedures done with this type of anesthesia, you may not be able to take over your own breathing again immediately. You may need a breathing machine for temporary life support, which may also increase the risk of complications.

Lung Tissue Removal

For someone with lung disease it is very important to decide before surgery whether they can tolerate the removal of any lung tissue, and if so, how much. For example, if you already have moderate COPD and are short of breath with ordinary activity, removing any good lung tissue at all may leave you completely disabled. If too much is removed, you may not be able to breathe well enough after surgery to come off the life-support breathing machine.

Because of these problems, lung doctors attempt to figure out before surgery how much lung function will be left after surgery. A decision has to be made whether the remaining lung function will be enough for you to get by on, and whether the surgery is worth the risk of your ending up a respiratory cripple.

Deciding about the effect of lung removal is done by performing a combination of tests. First, your breathing function is measured with spirometry, usually after you have used a bronchodilator to open your bronchial tubes as much as possible. The FEV_1 is calculated.

Then a test called a *lung scan* shows where in the lung the blood flow goes. A tiny amount of radioactive material is injected into your arm. How much blood flow goes to the right lung and how much to the left is calculated, and how much is in the lower half of the lung and how much in the upper. These two tests are put together to figure out what will happen after surgery.

For example, if you have lung cancer in the lower part of your right lung, to remove all the cancer requires removal of half the right lung. Your FEV_1 is 2.0 liters, 50% of expected. The lung scan shows that 50% of the lung function is in each lung. In the right lung, 50% of the function is in the lower half. This means that the surgeon would expect you to lose 25% of the total function by taking out the lower right lung, or half of the 50% on the right. After surgery, you would be expected to have an FEV_1 of 1.5 Liters (2.0 Liters X 75%). You should be able to breathe well enough after surgery that the cancer can be surgically removed.

On the other hand, suppose that your FEV_1 is only 1.0 Liter, 25% of expected. In order to remove the lung tumor, one half of the right lung has to come out. If the blood flow in the lung is going half to the right and half to the left, and in the right lung half of its flow is in the bottom, you will only have an FEV_1 of 0.75 Liters after surgery. This is probably not enough for you to breathe well enough to live independently. You would be a respiratory cripple. We would not perform the surgery and alternatives would be considered.

Importance of Surgery

If the surgery is only cosmetic and will not be important for your health or survival, do not have it done if it is at all risky. On the other hand, if you might die in the next several days without the surgery, you can accept risk. Some situations fall in the high-risk category.

For example, suppose your intestine is totally obstructed and no waste products will move through. If this is not corrected, you will die within days. If medical therapy fails, you may go to surgery knowing that there is some risk that you will end up on a mechanical ventilator or that you may die.

Many situations are not as clear cut. For example, if you have lung cancer, the surgeon may not be sure exactly how much lung will have to be removed to get all of the cancer out. If it is only necessary to take half the lung you may do all right, but if the whole lung needs to come out, you will not do well. In that setting, you and your doctors will have to decide together whether you will have as good a chance of survival and of breathing well enough to perform your usual activities. Because of the extent of the tumor and your poor lung function, the decision may be between treating the lung cancer with radiation or chemotherapy, or with surgery.

12 How to Make Life Easier

Sometimes, it's the little things that make big differences. These tips are a compendium of my own years of experience of living with chronic obstructive pulmonary disease. Many of them come from the people in the Cape COPD Support Group. None of the suggestions should be followed if they contradict your own doctor's prescribed treatment. Toward the end are some suggestions for being more comfortable with a cold or respiratory infection.

Tips

1. A hot beverage helps open clogged airways. If you are congested, have a cuppa' hot something, and see how quickly your breathing becomes easier. Soup, tea, coffee, hot water, hot chocolate—anything that steams.

2. Always, always rinse your mouth after using your puffer. This is most important with the corticosteroid inhalers. An alcohol-containing mouthwash to swish and spit is the most effective. This will help to prevent painful thrush, or rash, inside your mouth.

3. Carry your inhalers with you when shopping, socializing, or just walking. You never know when exertion will cause shortness of breath. A couple of puffs of Atrovent or Albuterol will help your breathing become more normal in minutes. Use those minutes to slow down, sit down, and rest.

4. Invest in MedicAlert to provide your medical history and prescribed medications by a toll-free telephone call, in case of emergency. The bracelet or pendant alerts the first responders (paramedics and hospital emergency room staff), briefly describes your illness or condition and gives the 800 number. This is especially wise if you are on supplemental oxygen or insulin, or if you have any severe allergies to drugs or anything else.

5. If you must make your bed, make up half of it (the side you aren't lying on) while you are still in the bed. The other half can be done more easily after you are up.

6. Although this has not been demonstrated scientifically, some people believe that dairy products increase sputum production. They believe that one should avoid cheeses and milk, and anything milk-based except yogurt if you are suffering from an infection in your lungs.

7. Sleep more comfortably with your head and back elevated. Use several pillows to prop yourself up from your mid-back to your head, or have your bed raised at the head by putting a wooden wedge under the mattress. It makes breathing easier.

8. If you are having trouble coordinating the movements to correctly use your inhalers, talk to your doctor about prescribing a spacer. Spacers like Inspirease™ and Aero Chamber™ are easy to use, and are pretty much fail-safe. You won't have the problem of leaving the medication in a puff inside your mouth, or worse, in your eyes if you really have bad aim or coordination. The spacer helps to deliver the medicine directly into your lungs, where it will be most effective.

9. Ask about the new powder inhalers. They are very easy to use. Many medicines are becoming available in a powder.

10. Take plenty of time in the shower. The moisture is good for your lungs, and you'll need extra time to rest a bit after shampooing and rinsing your hair. Rushing increases breathlessness.

11. And speaking of shampooing, the reason we get so exhausted when we wash our hair is that the arm movements required to apply lather, work it in, and rinse are aerobic exercise. Our lungs and heart are having to work harder. So shampoo when you start your shower, then bath, to have a brief respite from the aerobics, then rinse your hair, and finally your body.

12. Arrange your dishes and cooking utensils in your kitchen according to a list of most-often-used. Keep the everyday dishes and serving pieces no higher than eye-level in the cabinet, so that less physical strain is required to bring them out and put them away. Keep pots and pans nestled for easy access close to the stove, and where they won't require a knee-level search. This kind of planning helps you to conserve energy when cooking or cleaning up.

13. The old trick of setting things on the stairs to take on your next trip up is a good one. But make it a practice, for safety's sake, to clear the stairwell each time you go up.

14. Have at least one steamy bubblebath a week, over and above your daily showers. Consider it a time of relaxation and reflection. You can enjoy reading while you soak. This is good for your skin and your psyche. Breathe in that wonderfully soothing steam as you soak and daydream for awhile. Tune in to a classical radio station, and enjoy the luxury of relaxing.

15. For the ultimate in bath comfort, get yourself a tub pillow to rest your head on while reclining. They can be found at most cosmetic counters for less than $10. While you're there, treat yourself to a bottle of bath oil for your weekly soak, which will combat skin dryness that comes with aging.

16. If steam increases your coughing it may help to use your quick acting bronchodilator before your bath.

17. You probably qualify for handicap parking placards or license plates from the Division of Motor Vehicle Registration. Ask your pulmonary doctor to

apply for you, as it must be prescribed or officially requested by a doctor. When the ID arrives, use the privilege of parking closer to your destination. It saves countless steps, preserves energy, and helps you to arrive at your destination less breathless.

18. During the dry winter months, our homes and offices become too dry from the heat of furnaces and fireplaces. It is wise to operate a humidifier, at least in the room in which you sleep. This is especially important if you have electric heating. Invest in a small humidifier, and a thermostat that hangs on the wall to measure the humidity of the room.

19. Room humidity for lung disease should range between 40 and 60% at all times. You'll find that you'll suffer from fewer sinus infections, and that extra humidity is particularly helpful to oxygen users because oxygen by nasal cannula has a tendency to dry out the sinuses and cause painful nose polyps.

20. Never ever use a glycerine-based petroleum or gel to relieve nasal sores or sensitive nasal tissue. This can cause dangerous blistering. There are water-based gels on the market, available over the counter, which will do the same thing. Ayr is one of several brands.

21. Prepare a data card of your current medical information, and use a magnet to attach it to the front of your refrigerator. Paramedics and Emergency Medical Technicians are taught to look there for information in case of an emergency. On the card, list your illnesses, and all prescriptions that you take, with the amounts for each one. List, also, your primary care or pulmonary doctor's telephone number, and the name and number of your nearest relative or friend.

22. This may also be a good place to list the location of advance directives.

23. Anytime you are confronted with *stairs*, the nemesis of lung patients, use pursed-lip breathing. Inhale deeply through your nose, and as you exhale through pursed lips, take about three stairs up or down. Rest for a few seconds, take your next deep breath, and continue on the stairs for the length of your exhalation. Try to extend your exhalation to at least twice as long as your inhalation. You will arrive at the top of the stairs less winded and less tired with pursed-lip breathing.

24. Eat natural yogurt at least once a day. Yogurt helps to build up resistance to bacterial infections.

25. Buy unscented lotions, cosmetics, hair sprays and shampoos, laundry detergents and bath soaps. Strong scents can be irritating to the sinuses and lungs. Most lung patients develop a sensitivity to strong scents or smells. You'll probably find that you'll stop wearing perfume if you are a woman, and stop using colognes or after-shaves if you are a man.

26. Make one-dish meals, such as casseroles. Prepare large quantities and freeze in individual packages for future meals.

27. Don't get in a hurry while you are cooking. Pace yourself.

28. Use conveniences like microwave ovens and crock pots. Plan to do more baking than stove-top cooking. These meals may have less fat, are healthier and easier to prepare.

29. People with chronic lung disease may have low potassium levels. Low potassium levels can lead to electrolyte imbalance and even dehydration. If

your doctor confirms you have low potassium, discuss changes in your diet such as eating foods high in potassium every day: bananas, mushrooms, spinach, broccoli, oranges, tomato products, dried fruit, peanuts, winter squash, dry skim milk, potatoes, yams.

30. Try to get a little fresh air and light exercise before meals, particularly your evening meal. Both will sharpen your appetite.

31. Ask your oxygen provider to bring you a little cart on wheels that will hold your portable unit. When the portable is filled with liquid oxygen, it is too heavy to carry around by a shoulder strap. It is much easier to slip the unit into the cart, and then pull it behind you. My portable oxygen unit, the Cryogenic Stroller™, weighs about 10 pounds when filled.

32. The newer aluminum cylinders are much lighter. When used with an electronic demand valve they last about six hours.

33. Avoid carrying heavy items in your arms. Use a rolling cart for groceries, laundry, and equipment.

34. You'll probably feel more comfortable if you lean forward slightly when sitting for periods of time. This takes the strain of breathing off your neck and shoulder muscles.

35. Visualize for a good and comfortable feeling to control tension and to relieve stress. Use visualization as a mental escape whenever you find yourself in a difficult or painful situation.

36. Celebrate when you feel low. If you feel depressed or frustrated, find something to celebrate, and then, indulge yourself. Definitions of celebration and indulgence are different for everyone, but for me, it could be a new music CD, a book by a favorite author, a piece of chocolate fudge, a massage.

37. Alcohol is a depressant, so don't pour yourself a glass of wine or a highball or pop a beer if you are feeling depressed.

38. Remind yourself occasionally that you have limitations that are imposed by chronic illness. Ask for help when you need it. Fierce self-sufficiency may be more detrimental than accepting the fact that, once in a while, you need help.

39. Create opportunities for human contact. Reach out to people, and allow yourself to socialize as often as you can.

40. Join a Scrabble club at the Senior Center, or learn a new hobby, and find people to share the interest. Do not let yourself become isolated, or indefinitely introspective.

41. Morning seems a good time for a few warm-up exercises. Try making it a part of your daily ritual.

42. It is easier to do morning exercises while still in bed, before getting up. One of our support group members, Nina, relates her experience with daily exercise. She says that you'll feel better for having loosened up before you actively start your day.

43. As with any exercise program please clear this with your doctor before trying it.

44. She begins with repetitions of leg lifts, lying flat on her back, and does as many as are comfortable. The first type of exercise is simply bringing the

knee up toward the chest, alternating each leg. Then she does a few straight leg lifts, alternating legs.

45. Next, she does arm lifts and rotations.

46. If she feels well enough, she does a few sit-ups.

47. For stretching, she lies flat, then lifts one leg straight up and then lowers it to the opposite side of her body all the way till the toes touch the mattress, holding the leg as straight as possible. Raise it back up the same way it came down, and then lower it from a straight angle to the original flat position. Change legs, and repeat this great stretching exercise a few times on each side. Feel the stretch from your spine.

48. Then she sits up on the side of the bed and does repetitions of leg and arm lifts.

49. Another good stretch is to sit on the edge of the bed, swivel from the waist up to the left, allowing the left arm to move behind your seat and rest on the bed, and the right arm to go across your body to rest on the mattress to the left of your left hip. Hold this gentle stretch for a few moments, then switch to the other side. Repeat several times.

50. Allowing yourself plenty of time to do things is very important. You can still do many of the things you used to, although they may take longer.

51. Re-read your journal to find the times of day when you feel strongest and the most social. Schedule your activities accordingly, so that you can maximize your strength and energy.

52. When you have an important meeting or social commitment, plan to take a rest before time to go. Do this before your support group meeting, or doctor's appointment.

53. Allow yourself plenty of time, and a little extra, to make your appointments without rushing or hurrying. Getting there early is better than stressing yourself by pushing to make up lost time. Don't be robbed of your precious energy simply because you didn't start your shower on time, or didn't allow enough time to be punctual.

54. Allow yourself time each day for a little quiet reflection and rest. Just listen to soft music, or read a favorite book for a while. Small moments of privacy can be real power boosters in the middle of a stressed or pain-filled day. I fill those little oases of peace and quiet with mindful meditation, just allowing my mind to drain away the tensions and problems, and to ease my body with visualizations of quiet, tranquil pools of water, hearing birds sing and smelling flowers and freshly cut lawn. I like to visualize with the sensation of touch, too, trying to feel the warmth of the sun as I sit by an imaginary pool, by myself, with just the garden, the songbirds, and the fish in the pool for company. Privacy breaks like this are very restorative.

55. Pets are great companions, if you can have one or more, and have no allergies to them.

56. My two cats are characters, filled with personality and always entertaining, or just content to sit by my side as they run their purr motors.

57. A dog is as much company as any human being. My Connemara is my best friend, happy going with me wherever I go, and amazing me with her patience. She accompanies me to work each day, one of the big advantages

of living and working on Cape Cod; everyone here keeps their dog with them during the workday. She greets customers and their babies gently and with a friendly wag of her tail, in her role as mascot of Clambake Celebrations.

58. Dogs, particularly those which do not shed, like poodles or chihuahuas, are much less likely to cause allergic reactions than cats. If you have a lot of asthma trouble find out if cats are the cause.

59. One of my friends from the support group, Ellie, has a canary for a companion. You can always hear the cheery sound of that bird singing in the background, whenever you call Ellie on the telephone. If you live alone, having a devoted pet can save you from loneliness.

60. When a pet dies, grieving is natural. But replace it as soon as you can with another, possibly a different kind.

61. Change the filters in your heating or cooling units often. Take all steps that you can afford to make your home allergen-free.

62. For waiting in doctor's offices, or anywhere else, for about $10 you can acquire a tiny handheld poker or blackjack machine. They are battery operated, and provide hours and hours of entertainment as you try to beat the Vegas odds. They have a silence button you can press to play in complete silence, without disturbing anyone else in the room. You can find these little electronic wonders in many hardware stores, Radio Shacks and Walmarts.

63. Want to feel better? Hug somebody.

64. Get a copy of *Chicken Soup for the Soul*, by Jack and Mark Victor Hansen and use it. It's published by Health Communications, Inc.

65. Train yourself to tune in to your body, to listen to the signals your body sends. Learn the early symptoms of a developing infection to know when to call your doctor for help. Listen to your body's cry for rest, when it is needed. Recognize the wheezing sound of your airway when it starts to close up during an asthma attack, and be proactive about the early steps to control. Be sensitive to the signals. You can do all of this wisely and with common sense, without reacting like a hypochondriac.

66. Consider taking a daily multi-vitamin, and supplementary essential minerals. Good ones for COPD patients include anti-oxidants like selenium (which helps your body to use its oxygen more efficiently), vitamin C, and yeast-free chromium picolinate which helps to burn sugar, or boosts the effect of natural insulin.

67. Keep an open mind and be receptive to learning positive ways of controlling your illness.

Tips for Colds and Upper-respiratory Infections

Colds start as viruses, but can quickly become bacterial lung infections, which are even more dangerous with COPD. So here are some suggestions to get you through the rough times.

1. Drink plenty of liquids (preferably water, as it serves as a good expectorant to break up congestion in the chest).

2. Get more rest than usual. Short naps during the day will serve you well, and

help you to build resistance to infection.

3. Eat regular and nutritious meals. Many light meals during the day are better for you during a cold than heavy meals. They take up less room in your stomach and allow more room for your diaphragm to function, making breathing easier. Food provides energy for your body, and you'll need more energy during a cold or infection.

4. Take aspirin to relieve headache, achy body and fever. Wash it down with plenty of water.

5. Vitamin C is a good idea, especially if you can start taking it early, at the onset of the cold.

6. Make chicken soup a part of your daily diet for the duration of the cold. Research shows that good old-fashioned chicken soup helps if you have a cold. The hot liquid, or something in the soup fat is beneficial to people with stuffed up heads and rattling chests.

7. Hot soups or toddies raise body temperature and help to clear the nose.

8. Use disposable tissues, and wash your hands frequently.

9. Stay warm. Cold viruses thrive at lower temperatures.

10. With a stuffed-up nose, try draping a heavy towel over your head as you lean over to inhale steamy air from a bathroom sink full of hot water. After about 10 minutes you should be able to clear your nose with several good blows into your disposable tissue. This is a great relief for blocked sinuses too.

11. Do not take over-the-counter liquid cough suppressants without clearing it with your doctor. People with COPD actually *need* to cough to expel secretions in the lungs. It is better to get the phlegm and sputum up and out, than to let it stay there and become bacterial.

12. Don't eat dairy products (except yogurt) while you have a cold. Dairy products such as milk, cheese and ice cream are suspected of increased phlegm production. We have said "are suspected", so if dairy products don't bother you and you enjoy them, continue to eat them even with a cold or cough.

13. Don't give up on your exercise program while you have a cold. You won't feel much like exercising, but your body needs the muscle toning, even during a bout of sickness. And moderate exercise can help to jar secretions in the lungs loose for expulsion through coughs.

14. When you have a cold or other infection, do plan to rest after exercise.

15. Disinfect commonly used items, such as telephones, faucet handles and door knobs. Use anti-bacterial soaps to clean counter tops and to wash your hands. Stop the virus from spreading to other family members, from whom it may later rebound to you.

Renewal and Rediscovery

Chronic illness can take a terrible toll. Whether you are faced with chronic obstructive pulmonary disease, or lupus, or cancer, or muscular dystrophy, or even AIDS, each day presents a new set of demands or adjustments. We all seem to have some good days, but inevitably we must deal with bad days too. The so-called bad days may come with pain, or with other side effects, including depression.

Renewal is rediscovering aspects of yourself that allow you to feel content, even with the stress of illness, and to feel real joy in those moments of rapport with another or just with yourself.

Throughout the emotional process that goes with any chronic illness, you confront terror, loss, rage, all kinds of emotional pain. But when you are able to face the fear of the unknown and the pain of loss, you are on your way to achieving renewal. Finding the strength to face your dreads about illness helps you to not be overwhelmed.

Renewal is like finding yourself again. A self in new circumstances, with more constraints to handle, but with the tools to continue living regardless of radical change and loss of ability to do things you once loved. Renewal is not static, not passive. It is a dynamic attitude toward illness, born of all the struggles with COPD or any other long-term disability. You learn to set and reset your priorities in such a way that the capacities affected by illness no longer define you.

Hand-in-hand with renewal comes discovery, appreciating moments of respite and peace from the daily struggle to survive, savoring everyday events, and recognizing how deeply they influence you. Instead of focusing on what your illness makes you, focus on who you choose to be. It is entirely possible to be physically disabled without being emotionally handicapped.

Learn how to separate yourself from your illness. Be creative about adapting, and practice focusing on pleasure and the things that you can still do, rather than on your limitations and things you cannot do. Try to use some of your energy to help other people, and remain actively involved with living. Strive to not judge yourself too harshly. Accept your limitations, but never stop pushing the boundaries. Don't "Go gently into that good night". Live your life without regret and give yourself credit for the effort that it takes. Applaud yourself for being able-hearted. Look for the potential in tomorrow without trying to dictate exactly what tomorrow will bring. Know that, mostly, tomorrow can be taken in stride. The exquisite ability to be connected to yourself, to others, and to your environment outweighs physical limitations. Forgive yourself for what you are unable to do, and focus on the joys of rediscovering what makes you uniquely you. You'll find, within yourself, acceptance of your illness and the grace to continue. You'll rediscover self-esteem.

People with lung disease must eventually learn how to live with the physical limitations that are a part of the illness. Because of the demands of disability, we usually adapt to the boundaries on our activities fairly well, after a period of adjustment. We learn to manage daily living. But we seem to have a more difficult time adjusting mentally and emotionally to chronic illness.

Every person I know with COPD has had frequent bouts of depression after diagnosis, even with years and years of illness behind them. One of the reasons may simply be that COPD is a hidden disability, poorly understood or tolerated even by our closest friends and family.

Another reason for depression includes self-directed anger, because in the vast majority of cases, COPD is an illness that could have been avoided. If we had not smoked cigarettes, most of us would not now have a chronic illness that is progressive and incurable. It is hard not to be angry over the naive decision that we made to smoke when we were much younger.

Smoking cigarettes was, at the time, the "cool" thing to do. All of the movie stars and celebrities did it. Most of my peers puffed away. It was an easy way to rebel against parents and teachers. I think that learning how to smoke was the first thing I learned in college. And, did any of us really believe the warnings printed in small type on the cigarette packages? Did we feel vulnerable, or even mortal, at 18?

The anger, even rage, that comes from such self blame can fester, digging deeper and deeper into our psyches. And it can reappear days, months, even years after we think we have been able to exorcise most of the mental poison. Whether we're guilty of kicking ourselves or not, the damage we do to our self-esteem is corrosive.

Depression can also come from lack of independence, based on the inability to do for ourselves what we took for granted before we became ill. It hurts to have to rely on other people for help. It's hard for most of us to ask for assistance, when we have always been able to take care of our own needs. And it is doubly difficult when the people around us are unaware of our limitations.

The most valuable lesson I have learned about living with COPD, is that attitude plays as important a role as treatment. Good self-esteem can help us heal faster, cope with problems more effectively, and dramatically improve our quality of life. A positive attitude can be the first important step in our journey toward stability and emotional health. I believe that the mind has a powerful influence over the body, and that being negative shortens the lives of chronically ill people. The very essence of good psychological health is to maintain a positive attitude while knowing the facts and being realistic.

Thoughts on Death and Dying

People react differently to very bad news. And a diagnosis of COPD is certainly bad news. We have been advised that we have a chronic, so-far-incurable, usually-progressive illness. The lifestyle compromises that will eventually catch us may be overwhelming to consider. Our lives as we know them have just been shattered into fragments as sharp-edged as pottery shards. And somewhere in the shock of all that comes flooding in, thoughts of our own mortality will emerge.

For me, thoughts of dying were as unsettling as anything I had faced in my entire life. I was frightened, and I was shaken to the core. My energy and attention, which should have been focused on healing and overcoming the physical onslaught of the illness, were misdirected to unwanted thoughts about expiring from lung disease or its complications. And to concern for my family and friends.

I had to find ways to cope with the fear of an unknown, and unknowable, future. I learned over time that the best thing I could do for myself, whenever those thoughts of dying emerged, was to meditate for awhile, seeking a peaceful co-existence with the disease. The fear would pass, and my resolution to survive would become strengthened. As dark as those thoughts of death were, the comforting thing that I came to realize was that the anxiety that they caused was fleeting, and that I would naturally be able to work my way through them into the light again. But I had to work at it.

Putting the Fear of Death in Perspective

Unless you are severely ill and facing death within a very short time, the fear of death may be a form of anxiety—an expression of your sense of being helpless and your fear of losing control. Dr. Gary Paluba, a psychologist who counsels people in rehabilitation, recognizes this issue of losing control in many people with COPD (*Techniques to Control Dyspnea and Anxiety* on page 42). One source of anxiety is dyspnea. Another source of anxiety, as reported by Jo-Von, comes from confronting a difficult life situation and the recognition of one's mortality. Jo-Von's life felt 'shattered into fragments,' and she was overwhelmed by the multiple threats to her sense of control over her life.

In psychological perspective, the fear of dying is a form of anxiety based on the perceived loss of control. A psychologist may remind people who feel helpless, out of control, and anxious that they're probably going to live a long time, possibly another 20 years. He may tell them that to have a good quality of life they must take action to support their wellness—do their breathing exercises, do physical exercise, and take their medications.

Giving in to anxiety only intensifies your feelings of being out of control. However, you can learn to deal with your fears and reduce your anxiety by taking steps to regain control. You can do this by a realistic review of your reality—you are probably not actually going to die of COPD in the very near future. You can quickly gain your sense of control by doing your breathing exercises, or use meditation or other techniques like Jo-Von. Continue to learn about your disease and develop methods and plans for coping with daily life, and plan for unusual challenges like vacations. If you feel the urge to smoke as a response to anxiety, you may need to redouble your attention to smoking cessation. (See *Smoking* on page 105) You should consider getting professional advice for support in dealing with persisting fears and anxiety. And don't neglect to talk with your doctor, especially since some medications and medical conditions can cause a sense of anxiety.

Looking Out for Your Emotional Wellness

Learn to monitor your own emotional wellness. Not many people will be brave enough to tell us that we are slipping over the edge, but you can keep a close check on your own mental health by observing your effect on others, and by talking to loved ones and doctors, about your status. If you feel unable to manage the balancing process of mental stability by yourself, even with concentrated efforts to keep a positive attitude, then go to a psychologist for help. Your doctor or local hospital can make recommendations.

With that in mind, there are a number of steps we can take to protect ourselves from the stresses and strains of disability, or the stranglehold of depression.

Checklist for Controlling Your Life

The following suggestions can be used as a checklist for your own mental health. I urge you to review it frequently, daily if you have to, to bring a greater measure of control over your life, and to gain more assurance and confidence as you face each day. The list is brief, including commitments to ourselves that can keep us from spiraling downward. No one but you can do these things for you, so post it on your refrigerator and read it often.

❑ Keep learning about lung disease. Read articles, attend lectures, visit the library and do your own research. The more you know about your illness, the better you will be able to manage it.

❑ Take an active role in managing your illness. Become a good team member, and develop good communications with your pulmonary specialist. Ask questions when you don't understand or don't agree with prescribed treatment. Know your medicines, what they are for, and take them as directed.

❑ Participate in your support group. Don't be a bystander. Don't be passive. There is so much that we can learn from one another. Go to meetings. Absorb shared information. Contribute your own experiences. And most importantly, give support. Only people with the same illness can really support each other. Others, including well-meaning family members and spouses, can only guess.

❑ Maintain an exercise program. Even modest exercise, done consistently, is important in staying as fit as possible. Do what you can, and strive to increase your active exercise time.

❑ Be as active as you can possibly be, both mentally and physically. Fill your life with joy by engaging in activities that you love. Find hobbies that are interesting. Surround yourself with people who care about you, and with whom you can always find something to discuss. Getting out and about requires effort, but try to meet the challenge. Find events and activities that will enrich your soul.

❑ Keep your sense of humor. Laugh a lot, loudly, softly, chuckle, guffaw, or just plain ole' belly laugh. Give it your best shot.

❑ Feed the mind. If you like to read, allow yourself at least an hour a day to dive into a favorite book. If watching old classic movies brings you great happiness, keep a library of your own videos. Apply yourself to learning more and more about your illness, so that you'll know where to push the boundaries, and when to take risks.

❑ Feed the body. Don't neglect good nutrition. You need fuel to operate. Educate yourself and plan your meals to provide your body with the very best fuel. Nutrition is as important to a treatment program as medications and exercise.

❑ Feed the soul. Find the things that soothe your psyche and satisfy your soul, then write about them in your journal, so that you won't forget. Then go back to them for solutions as you need them, a place to go on the bad days, a place to go any time.

❑ Go in search of renewal and rediscovery each day. Make it your quest, an objective to look forward to each morning. Let positive emotional states lead you toward an accepting coexistence with your illness. Then you'll find peace.

13 Journal Samples

Here are some excerpts from a journal that I kept before I became ill, while I was on photographic safari in the jungles of Nepal.

The Himalayas Journal

I have seen a sight so significant, so relative to my perspective of life, that all other sights have paled.

I have felt the cold of a predawn on top of a mountain in the Himalayas, there to feel the chill change to a warm glow as the sun rose quickly over Annapurna.

How, indeed, can the snow glisten with such blinding intensity? The quiet takes my breath away as though sound can not be tolerated in such a setting.

Unknowingly I have committed it all to indelible memory. The feelings are of such magnitude that my words can not do them justice.

I am fortunate to have been there, and to be able to recall the experience in such vivid detail that I am again transported.

But I wish that I could hand you the scene, warm and moist as a raindrop, gently moved from my palm to yours.

I know of no other way to try to share it, my feelings for the Himalayas. I will answer their call again. Perhaps your shoulder will be next to mine as the clouds part to reveal the beauty of endless time.

The morning was covered by a soft, misty fog which put an automatic hushed feeling to the group. The silver-topped elephant grass sparkled with the heavy dew and bowed their high tips as if in deference to the beauty of the morning. It was cool, and the sounds of bush doves greeted us as we passed aboard our elephants.

The jungle loomed ahead, guarded first by the river, then by the elephant grass in such abundance that we literally could not see through it at times. As we entered the jungle the kai trees maintained a solitary salute, reaching their leafy fingers skyward to heights of a couple hundred feet.

What a tremendously peaceful feeling! This is what communing with Nature is all about. As we wind our way through the thick greenery, the mist begins to lift, and the sky turns from mauve to blue in a series of kaleidoscope dissolves. And the elephant plods along in her stoic way... incredibly sure-footed in this maze of trees and gullies and swampy fields.

I saw a leaf fall from a huge tree. It spiraled as it floated down to the ground. It was as though that leaf waited to join the earth until it had an audience. And I was an appreciative audience! It was a moment filled with magical qualities, good feelings. Mystical!"

Other Journals

I love reminiscing about precious times. My journal can take me back to the days when I could do things like mountain trekking, and riding elephants in exotic, faraway foreign lands. But it can also help me to keep things in perspective, and to view myself from a more distaff point of view, more abstractly, after the fact. For example, I wrote in my journal about an experience that I had a few months after I had been diagnosed. In hindsight, I realize that it was a time when I was grappling with the enormity of my own mortality.

Christmas season loomed ahead, and I was struggling with how to solve my gift list problem, absorbed as I was with the overwhelming aspects of adjusting to this illness. I decided to have a portrait done in a photo studio (something very unlike me, since I have always been far more comfortable behind a camera than in front of one). This, I thought, would be a gift I could give to both family and close friends... a framed picture of moi! I never acknowledged, even to myself, that this might be the last formal portrait I would ever have taken. Although I know that, subconsciously, the thought was what prompted me to this action. I was very sick at the time, and still very much in the throes of grieving for my own body which was betraying me.

So the sitting for the portrait was accomplished, even though I was self-conscious about the oxygen cannula, and removed it before the picture was taken. I didn't want my loved ones to remember me with a nasal cannula draped across my face! Now, to make a long story short, when proofs were ready, I selected the poses that I wanted, and ordered the number of prints that I would need for gifts, and chose the frames for the 5" x 7" prints. Done! I gave them out to the designated recipients during the holidays, and even felt very strange about giving out pictures of myself.

Much later, months after Christmas, I came across one of the prints in one of my family photo albums. I was astounded at what I saw! Shocked at the image that looked back at me from the photo, I examined the face closely to see what was wrong. And what I discovered, as I scrutinized my own image, was a face that mirrored the betrayal that I felt! The green eyes that looked back at me did not seem to be my own, but rather that of a victim of some horrible crime or attack; one who obviously felt deeply about being on the receiving end of such an attack, but who felt powerless to do anything about it! Strangely, by giving my friends and family a picture to remember me by, I had inadvertently put a victimized stranger's face into my own. For this person captured in the photograph was not me. The saddened face reflected only a stage of my adjustment to my illness. But, there it was, forever more, framed and staring back from the mantels and desks of nearly everyone I cared deeply about.

If my loved ones ever read this book, I think they'll know that this is my way of apologizing for sending them the look of "Poor pitiful Pearl" instead of my own, which is now steadfastly back on my own countenance. Maybe someday soon I'll have replacement photos done.

Here is another journal entry with memories of my childhood:

I grew up in a rural suburb of Dallas, where our street was the last barrier of houses before miles of wilderness. The neighborhood children all gathered at our favorite place to play, far from the prying eyes of grown-ups. We'd ride our bikes along the highway for about two miles, then leave the bikes in the ditch along the busy highway and walk inland from there for another mile or so. (This was back in a time when it was perfectly safe to leave our treasured bikes abandoned out in the open; no one would steal them. And no pervert would be waiting behind the trees! It was a simpler time.)

Our destination was a magical place that someone (who?) assigned the name of Pinnacle Peak. There were huge hills of white chalky rock, smoothed by the thousands of bare feet and the elements that ran over and over them. Trees grew in groves of deep shade, and punctuated the white hills like perfectly arranged subjects in a painting. A cold (even in hot, Texas summers) bubbling creek wound its way at the base of the hills, and provided us with fresh drinking water to go with the peanut butter and jelly sandwiches that we carried in our jeans pockets. (This was way before the days of those handy backpacks.) The sun warmed the rocky hills and gave us deliciously warm hard beds on which to lay as we shared our adolescent secrets and aspirations.

Pinnacle Peak was where I spent my summers, and even most Saturdays during the winter, if it wasn't too cold. There were never-ending adventures waiting there, and it was always a thrill to issue our Tarzan-sound call upon arrival, to see if one or more of our friends were already there, ready to answer with the same chest-thumping bellow! But it really didn't matter whether or not my playmates were there... I found just as much delight running over the hills, catching crawdads in the creek, studying the flora and fauna up-close-and-personal, and letting my imagination roam endlessly as I watched the thick clouds in the sky and listened to the song of mockingbirds. I was like a little wild thing myself, unrestrained, completely free, and drunk with life at the age of ten!

Even now, whenever I close my eyes and visualize Pinnacle Peak, I can feel the sun on my face, and hear children's laughter as it ricochets over the bald hills of chalk.

Another thought about journals... they make wonderful inexpensive (yet very personal) gifts! Give one to a friend, a sibling, or a grandchild. It's a lasting gift with unlimited promise and potential. But most importantly, give one to yourself to help you get through the difficult times. And to allow you to better remember the cherished times of your life.

Some Thoughts on My Own Battle

When my younger brother, Neil, returned from his service in Vietnam, he was a different person: quieter, withdrawn, somber, and didn't/wouldn't/ couldn't talk about what he had seen or done. There was pain and betrayal in his eyes, that has never quite gone away, even now.

I didn't understand. I was one of his biggest supporters, and was very proud of him. I thought he should be able to tell me war stories, the things that he went through. But I learned quickly not to push, and believed that eventually he would be able to talk to me about his service to his country. I knew that he was a paratrooper, and that he served in a Medical Evacuation Unit serviced primarily by helicopters. So I could imagine, to some degree, some of the atrocities that he had witnessed. Removing the badly mangled and torn bodies of other soldiers, some still alive, some not, had been his own hell, and had left indelible marks on his life.

After all these years, I now realize how difficult it would have been for my brother to verbalize the horror of Vietnam, even to me. And insult was added by people from his own country that ridiculed his participation, and had little empathy for those who served. The people who lived through it, brought it back in their hearts and their minds. Only those who were there would ever be able to fully understand how bad it was.

I only realized this after I began my battle with obstructive lung disease. No matter how well-intentioned our spouses, family, and close friends are, they can't know how we feel or what we are going through.

Walk in my shoes, if you want to feel my pain. Struggle for your next breath, if you seek to understand the panic of such moments. Come fight the next battle at my side, to know my enemy. But please don't expect me to try to explain it all to you, whenever you casually inquire how I am.

A co-worker told me about a woman who was an invalid that lived across the street from her husband's childhood home. As a boy, her husband used to see the lady occasionally seated in a wheelchair on the porch, her lap always covered with a robe. John never knew what was wrong with the woman, but still remembers his mother saying that the lady must have done something terribly wrong in her life for God to punish her like that! It is hard to imagine such ignorance today, although I know that it still exists. I've sensed such an attitude from a few people myself.

In my own experience I've observed the reluctance of some members of my family to accept the reality of my illness, and its ramifications. It seems very difficult for them to know the details of the diagnosis, or to understand the stress and strain of having to make the required lifestyle adjustments just to carry on.

14 Checklists, Measurements & Forms

Symptoms Checklist

Add your own symptoms to this list below. All of this will help your doctor to diagnose.

❑ Shaky

❑ Color and amount of sputum

❑ Heavy or tight chest

❑ Fatigue

❑ Fever

❑ Headache

❑ Appetite loss

❑ Cough

❑ Aching muscles

❑ Difficulty breathing, short of breath

❑ Temperature: _____°F _____°C

❑ Blood pressure: ____/___

❑ Distance walked at usual pace before stopping to rest: _____(feet or yards; city blocks; etc.)

❑ . . . .

❑ . . . .

❑ . . . .

❑ . . . .
❑ . . . .
❑ . . . .
❑ . . . .
❑ . . . .
❑ . . . .

Travel Preparation Checklist

Name_____

Physician: Dr. _____

Home Phone:(____)_____-_____

Phone No: (____)_____-_____

Address _____

Person(s) to Contact in case of an Emergency

_____ (____)_____-

_____ _____

(____)_____-_____

_____ (____)_____-

_____ Pharmacy: _____

❑ Do you have an ample supply of medicines for the trip?

❑ Did you pack your medicines in a carry-on bag?

❑ Did you pick up some extra inhalers?

❑ Did you arrange for antibiotics from your physician?

❑ Have you packed your respiratory care equipment?

❑ Did you pack all the necessary supplies?

❑ Do you have special meal requirements?

❑ Did you make arrangements for these?

❑ Are you required to get any special vaccinations?

❑ Have you packed appropriate clothing for the trip?

❑ Have you packed your Medicare or private insurance cards?

❑ Do you have proper identification?

❑ For emergency purposes do you have adequate cash, travelers checks, credit cards or can money be wired to you from your bank?

❑ Have you made arrangements for your mail in your absence?

❑ Do you need oxygen?

❑ Have you arranged for oxygen while on the airplane?

❑ Have you arranged for oxygen on the cruise?

❑ Have you arranged for oxygen when you arrive at your destination?

❑ If you use a concentrator, are there any special electrical requirements?

❑ Have you made arrangements for portable as well as home oxygen?

❑ Are you going to a higher altitude so you made need more oxygen? How much?

❑ What is your sleeping oxygen supply rate? _____ liters per minute

❑ What is your activity oxygen supply rate? _____ liters per minute

❑ How much extra oxygen will you need to use at your destination?
_____ liters per minute

❑ Oxygen Supplier:

_____

_____

_____

❑ What is the supplier's name, phone and address at your destination?

_____

_____

_____

_____

❑ What is the supplier's name, phone and address the first night en route?

_____

_____

_____

_____

❑ What is the supplier's name, phone and address the second night en route?

_____

_____

_____

_____

Body Fat Measurement

Today it is simple to measure body fat from skinfold measurements. Use a caliper and the tables provided below. After you have made skinfold measurements based on age and sex, make a few simple calculations. The figures and tables show sites for skinfold measurement.

Measuring with metric markings is easier and gives greater accuracy, so values in the tables below are in millimeters.

1 Secure a fold of skin and fat at a specific anatomic site then measure its thickness with calipers.
Use the correct locations indicated below for males and females.
Make the fold of skin and fat in the same direction as the fat normally distributes.
Pinch the fold firmly, but not too tightly.

2 Do not pick up underlying muscle in the skinfold.

3 Measure at least three times at each site for greater accuracy. Then add up the three measurements for the site and divide by three for an average.

4 Add the results of the two measurement sites together and use the "Percent Body Fat" table for your sex, to find your own body fat percentage.

5 To convert millimeters to inches, divide millimeters (mm) by 25.4 (number of mm in one inch). To convert inches to millimeters, multiply inches by 25.4.

Table 25: Where to take body fat measurements

Locations For Middle Aged Males	Locations For Middle Aged Females
Thigh, or front of the upper leg	Suprailiac, or just above the hipbone
Subscapular, or just below the wingbone of the back	Triceps, or back of the upper arm

Table 26: Percent body fat in women

Total mm	% Fat	Total mm	% Fat
20	9	90	27
25	11	100	28
30	13	110	29
35	15	120	30
40	17	130	31
45	18	140	32
50	20	145	32
55	21	155	33
60	22	165	34
65	23	180	35
70	24	185	36

Table 26: Percent body fat in women

Total mm	% Fat	Total mm	% Fat
75	25	200	37
80	26	210	38

Table 27: Percent body fat in men

Total mm	% Fat	Total mm	% Fat
15	15	60	31
18	16	63	33
21	17	64	34
24	18	69	35
27	19	72	36
30	20	75	37
33	22	78	38
36	23	81	39
39	24	84	40
42	25	87	41
45	26	90	42
48	27	93	43
51	28	96	45
54	29	99	45
57	30		

File of Life

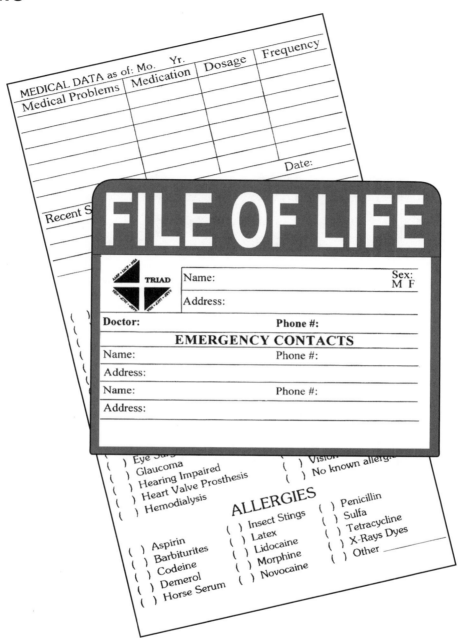

MEDICAL DATA as of: Mo.   Yr.

Medical Problems	Medication	Dosage	Frequency
			Date:

Recent S

FILE OF LIFE

TRIAD

Name: Sex:
                                             M F
Address:

Doctor: **Phone #:**

EMERGENCY CONTACTS

Name: Phone #:
Address:
Name: Phone #:
Address:

( ) Eye Sur
( ) Glaucoma   ( ) Vision
( ) Hearing Impaired   ( ) No known allerg
( ) Heart Valve Prosthesis
( ) Hemodialysis   **ALLERGIES**   ( ) Penicillin
                      ( ) Insect Stings   ( ) Sulfa
                      ( ) Latex   ( ) Tetracycline
( ) Aspirin   ( ) Lidocaine   ( ) X-Rays Dyes
( ) Barbiturites   ( ) Morphine   ( ) Other _____
( ) Codeine   ( ) Novocaine
( ) Demerol
( ) Horse Serum

15 Glossary

Acute: A situation or illness which occurs suddenly. Medically, may mean within a few hours or a few days.

Aerobic: In the presence of oxygen. Aerobic exercise is performed when ample amounts of oxygen are delivered to and used by the muscles.

Aerosol: A fine particle spray. Some inhaled bronchodilators are aerosols.

Aerosolize: Breaking liquids into small air-borne particles that can be inhaled.

Airway Obstruction: Narrowing, clogging or blocking of the air passages to or in the lung.

Allergy: Abnormal reaction to a stimulus called an allergen, such as pollen, shellfish, monosodium glutamate.

Alpha-1 Antitrypsin: Also termed alpha-1 antiproteinase deficiency. This is a protective material for the lung which is produced in the liver and transported to the lung. Deficiency occurs as a result of hereditary defects. Now there is alpha 1 replacement for this biochemical imbalance. However, the drug is very expensive.

Alveoli: Tiny sac-like structures at the end of the smallest bronchial tubes for the exchange of oxygen and carbon dioxide.

Anaerobic: Without oxygen. Anaerobic exercise is done with muscle cells lacking oxygen.

Antibiotic: A drug that kills or inhibits bacteria.

Antidepressant: A drug used to treat depression.

Anti-cholinergic: A drug that opens the bronchial tubes.

Apnea: The cessation (stopping) of breathing for a period of time, usually greater than 10 seconds while sleeping. Can be obstructive or the result of central brain dysfunction.

Arousal: Abrupt change from deep to lighter stages of sleep which may or may not lead to awakening.

Arteries: Large blood vessels that carry blood away from the lungs and heart.

Arterioles: Small, twig-like endings of arteries that lead to capillaries.

Asthma: A disorder of the bronchial tubes, making them too sensitive to irritants so that they narrow suddenly, causing difficulty breathing.

Asthmatic bronchitis: A type of bronchitis or bronchial irritation common with COPD. Causes asthma-like attacks, chronic cough, and mucus production.

Bacteria: Infectious organisms that may produce lung and other diseases.

Basal State: State of minimal metabolism in which the oxygen requirements of the body are at their lowest, resting level.

Beta receptor: A class of receptors (locks) for chemicals (keys) in cells throughout the body, including the muscles around the bronchial tubes. Beta receptors receive and respond to signals from other chemicals which the body releases and from some medicines. The receptors in the bronchial muscles control the size of the bronchial tubes, causing them to constrict or relax. A drug which is a *beta-2 agonist* will relax the airway, while a *beta-2 antagonist* will cause constriction.

BiPAP™ or **Bi-level PAP**: A positive airway pressure device used for breathing assistance in the case of severe lung disease, after lung surgery, or in the treatment of obstructive sleep apnea. Delivers small increases in inspiratory and expiratory pressure, to give relief to exhausted tissues, or to assist breathing with obstructive sleep apnea.

Blebs and Bullae: Localized destroyed portions of the lung that may occupy large portions of space within the lungs and that tend to crush normal lung tissue.

Blood Gas: A sample of blood, usually collected from the radial or brachial artery, in which oxygen, carbon dioxide, pH and other indices are measured.

Blood Gas Determinations: Measuring arterial blood gas.

Body Box: An airtight box which a person enters for measuring lung volumes. Provides medical data on the severity and type of lung compromise.

Booster: A single shot of a vaccine designed to increase the protective response from the original immunization.

Breath Sounds: Sounds heard by listening to the chest with a stethoscope, indicating movement of air within the lung.

Bronchi: Two main airways to and from the lungs. Singular is bronchus.

Bronchial Hygiene: Methods to rid the lungs and airways of irritants and retained secretions. The act of inhaling a bronchodilator, then inhaling moisture when needed, and making coughing efforts to expel materials for the airways.

Bronchiole: The smallest divisions of the bronchial tubes, less than 2 mm in size.

Bronchitis: Irritation of the lining of the bronchial tubes.

Bronchiectasis: Chronic dilation of bronchial tubes with secondary irritation and often infection in lower lung. Usually caused by a prior infection.

Bronchodilator Therapy: The act of using a bronchodilator (a medication that relaxes the airways and makes them larger).

Bronchoscopy: Inspecting and sampling of the airways.

Bronchospasm: Narrowing of the airways due to spasmodic contraction of the smooth muscles of the airway.

Bronchus: One of two main divisions of the trachea. Known as the right and left main stem bronchus. Bronchi applies to the two airways which result as the trachea divides.

Capillaries: The smallest of blood vessels which provide for the exchange of oxygen and carbon dioxide as well as other nutrients directly into the cells.

Cardiac Arrhythmia: An abnormal, usually irregular, heart beat.

Cardiac Arrest: Heart ceases to beat.

Cardiopulmonary System: Heart, blood and vessels, airways, lungs and the muscles that control breathing.

Cartilage: A ridged yet flexible supporting tissue somewhat similar to the structure of bone but not as rigid. Nose and ears are composed of cartilage.

Catarrh: Excessive production of mucus associated with a chronic cough.

Cholinergic: System that narrows the bronchial tubes in response to vagus nerve. Anti-cholinergic drugs prevent or reverse the narrowing.

Chronic: Illness which has been going on for some time. Medically, usually means months or years.

Chronic Obstructive Pulmonary Disease: Also known as Chronic Obstructive Lung Disease or Chronic Lung Disease. A broad term including one or more of emphysema, chronic bronchitis, bronchiectasis, and asthma.

Cilia: The hairlike structures that line the airways and beat rhythmically away from the lungs to propel mucus and foreign materials toward the mouth. The cilia are important defense structures and cleanse the lung of harmful debris. Destroyed by cigarette smoke.

Cor Pulmonale: Strain of the right side of the heart due to lung disease.

Cortisone: A steroid, a drug with important anti-inflammatory properties used to treat chronic and acute lung problems like bronchospasm and bronchial inflammation. Also essential for life and thus produced in the body in small amounts.

CPAP: Continuous Positive Airway Pressure. A device used to assist breathing, and in the treatment of obstructive sleep apnea capable of delivering small increases in inspiratory and expiratory pressure.

Decongestion: Reduction in the swelling of the nasal or lung air passages.

Desaturate: To lose blood oxygen.

Diffusion: Oxygen passing through walls of alveoli and blood vessels.

Diffusion Capacity: Ability of oxygen to pass through walls of alveoli and blood vessels, measured using a tiny amount of carbon monoxide.

DLCO: Lung diffusion for carbon monoxide. Used to measure the lung's ability to transfer oxygen between the alveolus and the capillary.

Diaphragm: The major respiratory muscle for breathing, and that separates the chest and abdomen.

Diuretics: A group of medications that cue the kidneys to increase removal of water and salt from the body.

Dyspnea: Shortness of breath or difficult breathing. Literally means bad breath.

Echocardiogram: Non-invasive imaging process to view heart function. A hand-held probe is placed on the chest of a prone person. Then a technician makes several pictures of the heart. Also takes pictures of babies in the womb.

Edema: Swelling caused by salt (sodium) and water retention.

Effluent: Streaming outward from any system, such as moisture from the nebulizer.

Electrocardiogram (EKG): A tracing of the heart's electrical activity. An important diagnostic tool that can reveal irregular heart beats, lack of oxygen to the heart muscle, heart strain, and medication effects.

Emphysema: Destruction or enlargement of alveolar sacs. Often caused by smoking.

Epithelia: Lining cells of bronchial tubes.

Expectorant: A drug that improves the thinning and removal of secretions from the respiratory tract.

Exacerbation: Worsening of the severity of a disease.

Exhalation: Breathing air out of the lung.

Expiration: Exhaling air from the lungs. Also means to die.

Genetic: Inheritable features passed from parents to child, such as color of eyes and hair, and certain diseases.

Glandular: A type of cell which makes a liquid and releases it to the body, like mucus in the nose.

Heart Failure: Inability of the heart to circulate blood efficiently. When the heart is strained it has decreased ability to pump blood. Can be treated with a variety of drugs.

Hemoglobin: A chemical carried in the blood by red blood cells, and which can take up oxygen and efficiently deliver it to other cells and tissues. Colors blood red.

Hemorrhage: Escape of blood from a blood vessel in some part of the body.

Humidification: Moisturizing. For supplemental oxygen delivery, bubbling the oxygen through a bubble humidifier to increase the water content before breathing.

Hyperventilation: A state in which abnormally fast and deep respirations result in reduced carbon dioxide in the blood. May cause dizziness or fainting.

Hypoventilation: Not enough air entering and leaving the lungs to bring oxygen to the tissues and eliminate carbon dioxide.

Hypoxemia: Not enough oxygen in the blood.

Hypoxia: Lack of oxygen.

Inflammation: Irritated, reddened and swollen tissue.

Inflammatory Cells: Cells released by the body to attack bacteria or other invaders, or in response to cigarette smoke. May themselves damage lung tissue.

Influenza: A viral infection, usually occurring in the winter and causing high fever and, frequently, breathing problems. Also called the flu.

Inspiration: Movement of air into the lungs.

Irritant: Any noxious agent that may cause damage to the lungs.

Ischemic Heart Disease: Heart disease from restricted blood supply due to obstruction in the blood vessels. The usual cause of heart attacks and angina.

JCAHCO: Joint Commission for Accreditation of Health Care Organizations

Lymph Gland or **Node**: Pea-sized glands that contain lymph. These glands are important defense mechanisms against infection.

Lymphatic Channels or Ducts: Delicate vessels that move lymph fluid to the lymph glands.

Macrophage: Scavenger cells found in the blood that have the ability to consume and carry away foreign materials. Also have the ability to move to the lung and fight infection and chronic irritation.

Medulla: Located at the base of the brain, nervous center for respiratory functions.

Metabolism: Consumption of oxygen and nutrients to produce energy and maintain living tissue.

Microgram: A unit of measure in the metric system. It is one-millionth of a gram.

Mucolytic Agent: A drug that can dissolve mucus. Lytic means to destroy.

Mucus Glands: Glands that provide mucus for cleansing the lungs and respiratory system. These glands are enlarged in chronic bronchitis.

Nares: Openings in the nasal cavities or nostrils.

Nebulizer: A device that takes a liquid and breaks it into tiny droplets of a size that can be inhaled into the lung.

NonREM Sleep: A nonuniform series of four stages of sleep which occur early in the night and are characterized by the absence of movement and slow brainwave activity. NonREM sleep generally comes before the first REM period.

Oximeter: A device which measures the amount of oxygen associated with hemoglobin.

Oxygen Transport: Movement of oxygen to tissues. A function of the lungs and the circulatory system.

Pathologic: Abnormal body functions.

Pedometer: A device that measures walking distance. In appearance it is similar to a watch and functions by measuring distance covered through the movement of walking.

Phlebotomy: Removal by needle of blood from the body.

Phlegm: Glutinous or sticky mucus.

Physiologic: Normal body functions.

Pleura: The thin membrane that encases the lungs and lines the chest cavity.

Pneumonia: An infection of localized areas within the lung. A common infection in patients with COPD. Caused by a variety of organisms, including bacteria and viruses, and by some chemicals.

Pneumococcal Vaccine: A vaccine given to prevent pneumonia caused by a common bacteria, the pneumococcus.

Pneumothorax: Collapse of a lung caused by air that leaks out of the lung and collects between the lung and the chest wall, causing chest pain and labored breathing.

Polysomnogram: Name for a sleep study.

Postural Drainage: Positioning the body so that gravity can assist in draining mucus from the lungs.

PRN: Pro re na 'ta. According to circumstances.

Prophylactic Treatment: Prevention. Also called prophylaxis.

Prostaglandins: A group of fat-derived chemicals involved in the regulation of a number of body functions.

Protuberant: Sticking out.

Pulmonary Function Test: Measures the degree of damage to the lungs. The most common tests use a spirometer to measure the ability of the lung to move air into and out of the lung.

Pulse: Throbbing or beats felt in arteries of the body when the heart contracts.

Pulse Oximeter: Non-invasive device that measures the oxygen in the blood through a clip on finger, ear, or nose and a high-intensity light. Pulse refers to the measurement of oxygen when the pulse is sensed.

Rapid Eye Movement: A stage of sleep in which dreaming is associated with mild involuntary muscle movements. Adults cycle in and out of REM at about 90-minute intervals. REM occupies 20% of total sleep time.

Red Blood Cells: Cells that contain hemoglobin, an iron compound necessary for transporting oxygen.

Resistance: Impediment to flow in or out of the lungs.

Respiration: Taking air into and out of the lungs, and use of oxygen at the cell level.

Respiratory Center: An area of the brain (medulla) that controls respiration or breathing. This area is stimulated by a lack of oxygen or by too much carbon dioxide.

Respiratory System: The system that breathes gases in and out of the body, including airways, lungs, bones and muscles.

Respiratory Failure: The lungs cannot supply enough or any oxygen to the body nor remove carbon dioxide. May be acute or chronic. Not likely to be curable if chronic.

Sedative: A drug designed to promote sleep or relaxation.

Sleep Fragmentation: Interruption of a sleep stage by awakening or appearance of another sleep stage.

Sleep Hygiene: Conditions and practices that promote effective and continuous sleep, such as regular bedtime and arise time, restriction of alcohol and coffee.

Sleep Latency: Time measured from lights out or bedtime to actually falling asleep.

Sleep Study: An overnight laboratory study to evaluate different physiologic aspects of sleep. Usually includes extensive monitoring and visual observation.

Somnolence: Excessive sleepiness. May result from drugs or from severe states of respiratory failure during which the lungs are not providing enough oxygenation and carbon dioxide removal.

Spirometer: Device to measure breathing capacity.

Sputum: Mucus or phlegm that comes out of the respiratory track.

Sternum: Breastbone.

Stethoscope: Device used to listen to heart and lung sounds.

Tapered: Gradually decreasing medication dosage.

Tenacious: Secretions that are thick, sticky, and difficult to remove.

Therapeutic Level: Curative level. Level of medication that should cure.

Thorax: The muscular and bony part of the chest.

Thrush: Common fungal infection.

Toxicity: Undesirable result of drug use.

Trachea: Main airway or wind pipe supplying the lungs.

Tracheostomy: Surgical procedure providing an opening into the windpipe or trachea.

Tracheostomy Tube: A plastic or metal tube placed in the trachea through a small surgical opening.

Training: Exercise, as in weight training, aerobic training.

Tranquilizer: A sedative-like medication used to reduce anxiety.

Trans-tracheal Catheter: A small catheter or tube inserted through a small hole in the windpipe to provide long-term oxygen delivery.

Treadmill: Device used to walk. Some treadmills have both speed and elevation adjustments that allow the amount of work to increase.

Vaccine: An injection that may stimulate an immune response. The immune response may be protective against a natural infection or lessen its severity.

Veins: Large blood vessels that return blood from the body and the lungs and to the heart.

Ventilation: The act of breathing or moving air into and out of the lungs.

Ventilator: Breathing machine used to treat respiratory failure.

Virus: A group of highly infectious agents that cause a variety of illnesses. Viruses are not killed by most antibiotics.

Wheeze: Whistling sound of air entering or leaving the lungs. Can be a sign of muscular spasm in the bronchial tubes.

White Blood Cells: Cells which usually fight infection. The white cell count usually increases with infection due to wars with bacteria.

16 Bibliography

Access Travel: Airports, Item 570-C, Publication from the Consumer Information Center, Pueblo, CO. 81009

Adjustments To A Chronic Illness by Dr. Greg Franchine, National Jewish Hospital for Immunology and Respiratory Medicine, 1994.

After The Diagnosis; From Crisis to Personal Renewal for Patients with Chronic Illness, by JoAnn LeMaistre, Ph.D., Ulysses Press, Berkeley, CA., 1995.

Allergy and Asthma Information Center & Hotline, P.O. Box 1766, Rochester, NY 14603. Tollfree: 1-800-727-5400.

The American Medical Association Encyclopedia Of Medicine, Medical Editor Charles B. Clayman, M.D. Published by Random House New York. This is an A-to-Z reference guide to over 5,000 medical terms including symptoms, diseases, drugs and treatments.

Being Close, Understanding Asthma, Understanding Emphysema, Nocturnal Asthma, Management of Chronic Respiratory Disease, Understanding Allergy, and many other pamphlets; National Jewish Medical and Research Center, 1400 Jackson Street, Denver, CO 80206. Telephone (303) 388-4461.

Breathe Right Now: A comprehensive guide to understanding and treating the most common breathing disorders; Smolley, Lawrence A. and Debra F Bruce; 1998; New York: WW Norton.

Breathing Disorders: Your Complete Exercise Guide. 1993. Neil G. Gordon, Champaign, IL: Human Kinetics

Breathing Disorders Sourcebook. 1998. Adams, Francis. V, Lincolnwood, IL: Lowell-NTC/Contemporary

Breathin' Easy: A guide for travelers with pulmonary disabilities, Gorby, Jerry

Chicken Soup For The Soul, 101 Stories To Open The Heart And Rekindle The Spirit, written and compiled by Jack Canfield and Mark Victor Hansen, Health Communications, Inc., Publishers

The Chronic Bronchitis and Emphysema Handbook. 1990. Francois Haas and Sheila Sperber Haas. New York: Wiley Science Editions

Coordinating Breathing With Body Movements, from the Pulmonary Rehab Program at The National Jewish Medical and Research Center, 1400 Jackson Street, Denver, CO 80206. Telephone (303) 388-4461.

Disease Management of COPD With Pulmonary Rehabilitation, Brian L. Tiep, CHEST 1997; 112:1630-56

Enjoying Life With Chronic Obstructive Pulmonary Disease. 1995. Petty, Thomas L. and Louise M. Nett, Cedar Grove, N.J.: Laennec.

Enjoying Life With Emphysema. 1987 Petty, Thomas L. and Louise M. Nett, Philadelphia: Lea & Febiger

Environmental Control And Information About Allergies And Asthma: Asthma & Allergy Foundation of America, 1125 15th St. N.W., Ste. 502, Washington, DC 20005. Tollfree: 1-800-727-8462.

Equal Partners: A Physician's Call for a New Spirit of Medicine. 1995. Heymann, Jody, M.D. Little, Brown & Company.

Essentials of Pulmonary Rehabilitation (In three parts); Pulmonary Education and Research Foundation, POB 1133, Lometa CA 90717

Full Catastrophe Living, Using the Wisdom of Your Body and Mind to Face Stress, Pain and Illness. 1990. Jon Kabat-Zinn, Ph.D. Dell Publishing. The basic program of the Stress Reduction Clinic at The University of Massachusetts Medical Center.

Good If Not Great Travel With Lung Disease, 1999. Petersen, Phil. Charlotte, NC: Raven POB 242275 Charlotte NC 28224-9798; Telephone (888) 552-2477 <http://www.oxygenbook.com>

Good If Not Great Living With Oxygen, 1993. Petersen, Phil. Charlotte, NC: Raven POB 242275 Charlotte NC 28224-9798; Telephone (888) 552-2477 <http://www.oxygenbook.com>

The Healing Power Of Doing Good. 1991 Allan Luks with Peggy Payne. Ballantine Books. A book about the spirit of giving, and its healing power.

Healthy Breathing, National Jewish Medical and Research Center, 1400 Jackson Street, Denver, CO 80206. Telephone (303) 388-4461.

Heaven's Coast: A Memoir. Doty, Mark. New York:Harper Collins, 1996

Help Yourself to Better Breathing, About Oxygen Therapy at Home, and *Around the Clock with COPD;* pamphlets from American Lung Association, 1740 Broadway, New York, NY, 10019.

How To Start A Peoples' Medical Library, and *The Planetree Health Catalog* which offers many excellent home medical reference books. Planetree Health Resource Center, A Division of California Pacific Medical Center, 2040 Webster Street, San Francisco, CA. 94115. Telephone (415) 923-3680

*Information Provider.*The National Organization for Rare Disorders, New Fairfield, CT.

Keep On Keeping On: Emphysema and Me...and You, Too, Dunham, William B. Annapolis: Anne Arundel Medical Center. 1996

Letters from Tom by T. L. Petty; as printed in the *Second Wind Newsletter*; Presbyterian St. Lukes Medical Center, 1719 E 19th Ave, Denver CO 80218.

Living Beyond Limits, New Hope and Help for Facing Life-Threatening Illness. 1993. David Spiegel, M.D. Times Books, Random House.

Living Well with Chronic Asthma, Bronchitis, and Emphysema: A Complete Guide to Coping with Chronic Lung Disease. 1991. Myra B. Shayevitz, Berton R. Shayevitz and the Editors of Consumer Reports Books. Yonkers, NY: Consumer Reports Books.

Lung Disease Data, 1995. The American Lung Association. 1740 Broadway, New York, NY 10019. Telephone 1-800-586-4872. <http://www.lungusa.org>[1].

The Magic Shop: An Imaginative Guide to Self Healing, Graham, Helen, 1992.

New Horizons For The Air Traveler With A Disability, Item 573-C, Publication from the Consumer Information Center, Pueblo, CO. 81009.

Newsletter of the Cape COPD Support Group, c/o Clambake Celebrations, 1223 Main Street, Chatham MA 02633

Nursing Drug Handbook, published by Springhouse Corporation, newest version.

Phantom of the Night: overcome sleep apnea syndrome and snoring—win your hidden struggle to breathe, sleep, and live. 1998. T.S. Johnson and J. Halberstadt, Onset: New Technology Publishing.

Phantom of the Night: overcome sleep apnea syndrome and snoring—win your hidden struggle to breathe, sleep, and live. 2000. T.S. Johnson, J. Halberstadt, and W. Broughton, Onset: New Technology Publishing.

Physicians' Desk Reference: PDR 52 Edition 1998, Montvale NJ: Medical Economics Company, 1998

Prevention, a magazine published by Rodale Press. Rodale Press is a source for reference books and other printed materials on many diseases and illnesses, and on wellness.

Priorities, the Allergy and Asthma Relief Catalog. Products to help protect you from allergens, asthma triggers and chemical toxins. Information about ways to safeguard your home and to make it allergen-free. Call 1 800 553-5398 to request a free catalog. By email: getrelief@priorities.com. <http://www.priorities.com>.

The Pulmonary Paper: Dedicated to Respiratory Health Care, POB 877, Ormond Beach FL 32175, 1-800-950-3698; $17.95/year; belyea@aol.com, <http://www.pulmonarypaper.org>

Second Wind Newsletter: Pulmonary Education & Research Foundation; POB 1133; Lomita CA 90717-5133; $20/year

Shortness Of Breath, A Guide To Better Living And Breathing. 1996. Ries, Andrew L.MD, MPH; Kenneth M. Moser, MD; Patricia J. Bullock, RRT, RCP; Trina M. Limberg, BS, RRT, RRP; Roseann Myers, RN, BSN; Dawn E. Sassi-Dambron, RN, BSN; Jamie B. Sheldon, PT, Fifth Edition,. St. Louis, MO: Mosby.

Sick Lungs Don't Show; pamphlet from Family Support Group of the American Lung Association of Hennepin County, 1829 Portland Ave., Minneapolis, MN 55404. Telephone (612) 871-7332, Fax (612) 871-9441.

---

1. References to the URL or universal resource locator address system of the World Wide Web are set off by angled brackets, thus: <http://>.

Other Resources

Organizations

Allergy & Asthma Information Center & Hotline, P.O. Box 1766, Rochester, NY 14603. 1-800-727-5400. Information on environmental control, allergies and asthma.

Alpha1 National Association, 8120 Penn Ave South Suite 549, Minneapolis, MN 55431-1326, 1-800-521-3025 <http://www.alpha1.org>[1] "A non-profit, membership organization, dedicated to improving the lives of individuals and their families affected by alpha1-antitrypsin deficiency."

Alpha One Foundation (Alpha-1 antitrypsin) 2937 S.W. 27th Avenue, Suite 302 Miami, Florida 33133 Toll Free: (888) 825-7421, 305-567-9888, Fax 305-567-1317 <http://www.alphaone.org> "The vision of the organization is to advance the means to control and cure A1AD and to improve the quality of life for those with the disorder. "

American Association for Cardiovascular and Pulmonary Rehabilitation, 7611 Elmwood Avenue, Suite 201, Middleton WI 53562. 608-831-6989 <http://www.aacvpr.org/>

American Cancer Society, 1-800-ACS-2345 <http://www.cancer.org/>

American College of Chest Physicians, 3300 Dundee Road, Northbrooke IL 60062-2348. <http://www.chestnet.org/>

American College of Sports Medicine, 1740 Broadway NY, NY 10019-4374401 West Michigan St. Indianapolis, Indiana 46202-3233

American Heart Association, National Center, 7272 Greenville Avenue, Dallas, Texas 75231 <http://www.amhrt.org> Customer Heart and Stroke Information 1-800-AHA-USA1, Women's Health Information 1-888-MY-HEART

---

1. References to the URL or universal resource locator address system of the World Wide Web are set off by angled brackets, thus: <http://>.

American Lung Association, 1740 Broadway, New York, NY 10019. 1-800-LUNG-USA, 1-800-586-4872. <http://www.lungusa.org>.

American Lung Association of Hennepin County, 1829 Portland Ave., Minneapolis, MN 55404. (612) 871-7332, Fax: 612-871-9441.

American Thoracic Society, Medical Section of the American Lung Association, 1740 Broadway, New York, NY 10019, 212-315-8700, Fax: 212-315-6498

Asthma & Allergy Foundation of America, 1125 15th St. N.W., Ste. 502, Washington, DC 20005. 1-800-727-8462. Information on environmental control, allergies and asthma.

Better Breathers Club: Check with your local hospital; the American Lung Association has local groups that can direct you, call them or try their web site.

Cape COPD Support Group, c/o Clambake Celebrations, 1223 Main Street, Chatham, MA 02633

Healthy Resources™ provides access to discussions and support among people with COPD, news and information, and products. It includes the web page for this book and is a service provided by New Technology Publishing, Inc. <http://www.HealthyResources.com>.

Department of Environmental Protection (Massachusetts only) 1-800-882-1497. Ozone and pollen count, air quality rating, updated twice daily.

MedicAlert Foundation International, Turlock CA 95381-1009, 800-ID-ALERT. System to provide emergency medical information by telephone about subscribers who carry or wear an identification bracelet or necklace.

The National Jewish Medical and Research Center, 1400 Jackson Street, Denver, CO. 80206, 303-388-4461. 1-800-222-LUNG. Call the National Jewish Medical and Research Center toll free line for connection to a nurse or respiratory therapist, or to request information from a doctor. <http://www.njc.org/njc.html>

National Oxygen Travel Service (NOTS), Dayton, Ohio.

National Emphysema Foundation, Sreedhar Nair-M.D., Chest Medicine, Norwalk Hospital, Norwalk, CT 06856 Education and research. <http://www.emphysemafoundation.org/> e-mail Address : gary@emphysemafoundation.org

Nutrition Screening Initiative, 1010 Wisconsin Ave. NW, Suite 800, Washington, DC 20007, 202-625-1662; <http://www.aafp.org/nsi> See *The Nutrition Checklist* and *Strong & Healthy.*

Pulmonary Education and Research Foundation A Guiding Program for Enjoying the Breath of Life. Education, research, information. Second Wind Newsletter. PERF P.O. Box 1133 Lomita, California 90717-5133, 310-539-8390 <http://www.perf2ndwind.org/>

Planetree Health Resource Center, A Division of California Pacific Medical Center, 2040 Webster St., San Francisco, CA. 94115. 415-923-3680. Data search, research.

University of Texas Health Center, US 271 at SR 155, Tyler TX 75708. 903-877-3451

Online Information

Airwaves, an Internet newsletter for people with COPD
<http://www.thebreathingspace.com>[1]

Allergy Control Products, Inc. 800-422-DUST; <www.allergycontrol.com>

Alpha1 National Association, <http://www.alpha1.org>

Alpha One Foundation <http://www.alphaone.org>

American Association for Cardiovascular and Pulmonary Rehabilitation, <http://www.aacvpr.org/> See the online "Program Directory" listing over 1,100 rehabilitation programs, including certification of qualified programs. Programs must pay for their listings, therefore there may be gaps in coverage.

The American Lung Association, 1740 Broadway, New York, NY 10019, 1-800-586-4872. <http://www.lungusa.org>

Bill Horden's web site <http://members.aol.com/SOBnSA/home.index.html>

Breathin' Easy Travel Guide: Web site in affiliation with the AARC; lists oxygen suppliers throughout the United States. Suppliers must pay for their listings, therefore there may be gaps in coverage. <http://www.oxygen4travel.com>

Healthy Resources™ provides access to discussions and support among people with COPD, news and information, and products. It includes the web page for this book and is a service provided by New Technology Publishing, Inc. <http://www.HealthyResources.com>.

National Allergy Supply, Inc., 800-522-1448; <www.nationalallergysupply.com>

National Emphysema Treatment Trial (NETT), supported by the National Heart, Lung, and Blood Institute (NHLBI), the Health Care Financing Administration (HCFA), and the Agency for Health Care Policy and Research (AHCPR); Evaluation of Lung Volume Reduction Surgery for Emphysema <http://www.nhlbi.nih.gov/nhlbi/lung/nett/lvrsweb.htm>

National Lung Health Education Program (NLHEP), in collaboration with National Heart, Lung, and Blood Institute; National Cancer Institute; Amercan Thoracic Society; American College of Chest Physicians; American Association for Respiratory Care. email: <NLHEP @aol.com> <http://nlhep.org>

Phantom Sleep Resources™ is a service provided by New Technology Publishing, Inc. to help you overcome sleep apnea, snoring & other sleep problems. <http://www.HealthyResources.com> or <http://www.newtechpub.com>

Pulmonary Education and Research Foundation A Guiding Program for Enjoying the Breath of Life. Education, research, information. Second Wind Newsletter. email: <perf@pacbell.net> <http://www.perf2ndwind.org/>

Priorities, the Allergy and Asthma Relief Catalog. Products to help protect you from allergens, asthma triggers and chemical toxins. Information about ways to safeguard your home and to make it allergen-free. Call 1-800-553-5398 to request a free catalog. By email: getrelief@priorities.com. <http://www.priorities.com>.

---

1. References to the URL or universal resource locator address system of the World Wide Web are set off by angled brackets, thus: <http://>.

About the Authors & Contributors

The Authors

Rick Carter, Ph.D. MAS, MBA is Professor of Medicine and Physiology at the University of Texas Health Center, Tyler, Texas, a center for excellence in chest diseases. Dr. Carter has extensive clinical, research, and administrative experience in the areas of exercise physiology and pulmonary rehabilitation. With nearly 20 years experience in assisting patients (heart and lung) in rehabilitating functional status and improving quality-of-life, he is now the principle investigator of a large rehabilitation trial funded by the National Institutes of Health through the Agency for Health Care Policy Research. He has published many scientific papers, in addition to presentations at national and international professional meetings. He continues to explore new opportunities for helping patients improve their functional ability and quality-of-life.

Brooke Nicotra, M.D. is retired Professor of Pulmonary and Critical Care Medicine at the University of Texas Health Center, Tyler, Texas, a center for excellence in chest diseases. Dr. Nicotra has more than 25 years' experience caring for patients with pulmonary disease and has published over 40 peer-reviewed papers in pulmonary medicine. She has passed specialty Boards in Internal Medicine, Critical Care Medicine, and Pulmonary Medicine. During her professional career she has encouraged patients to take an active role in their own care. She is an accomplished clinician, teacher, and clinical investigator. Above all she remains committed to the caring and individualized approach to medicine.

Jo-Von Tucker owns and manages *Clambake Celebrations*, a national mail-order speciality food company located in Chatham, Massachusetts. She is a founder and the coordinator of the *Cape COPD Support Group,* and a COPD patient. She is the recipient of more than 400 international awards of excellence in her direct marketing career. Her photograph appears on the cover. She has survived with COPD for ten years so far and looks forward to many more productive years.

Contributors

Thomas Petty, M.D. has had a distinguished career in pulmonary medicine. A pioneer in COPD treatment and education, he continues his work to educate physicians and the public to the value of early diagnosis and intervention to reduce the impact of COPD. He is the author of books on COPD for the patient, as well many scientific books and papers. He is Professor of Medicine, University of Colorado Health Sciences Center, and Chairman, National Lung Health Education Program (NLHEP). The NLHEP is a new national health care inititive aimed at involving primary care physicians in the early diagnosis and treatment of COPD and related diseases. He lives and practices in Denver, Colorado.

Dr. Brian Tiep, M.D. is one of the pioneers of specially-developed pulmonary rehab programs for COPD treatment. A noted speaker and lecturer in pulmonary diseases, he is Associate Professor of Medicine at Western University Health Sciences in Pomona, California. As Medical Director of the Pulmonary Care Continuum, Dr. Tiep is engaged in training physicians and other health care professionals for establishing and managing pulmonary rehabilitation programs for COPD. He seeks to make pulmonary rehabilitation available to all with continuing reinforcement as part of their relationship with their own physician. In addition to authoring many papers on rehabilitation for patients with pulmonary disease, he has played a role in developing innovative treatments and devices. He is a strong proponent of the roles of exercise, fitness, education, and mental attitude in restoring quality of life.

Richard T. Knowles, Ph.D. is a psychologist in private practice and affiliated with the Pulmonary Care Continuum, helping to develop programs for COPD. He has done extensive consulting in a variety of institutions and organizations, including helping people to deal with and manage stress, drugs, suicide, and death.

Other Contributors

Numerous patients and professionals read one or more drafts of this book and made insightful and helpful comments. The authors are grateful to each of them.

Hank Kite, whose lifelong strength and leadership was always available to encourage and guide others, advised on the development of this book. Although his personal struggle with COPD has ended, his spirit of encouraging others to equal strength and courage is memorialized in this book.

Respiratory therapy

Ron Corbett, a respiratory therapist at Cape & Islands Oxygen Supply, in Hyannis, Massachusetts, provided helpful information and read several drafts of the chapter on supplementary oxygen. Cape & Islands Oxygen Supply also provided the loan of the Oxymatic portable system for Jo-Von Tucker to use for the cover and other illustrations.

Sleep medicine

Gila Lindsley, PhD kindly reviewed and helped revise the material on sleep apnea. Dr. Lindsley is a diplomate of the American Board of Sleep Medicine and has a clinical practice, SleepWell™, based in Lexington, Massachusetts.

Psychology of stress management

Gary V. Paluba, PhD kindly reviewed the manuscript and made helpful contributions to the discussion of anxiety, depression, fear of death, and the use of pursed lip breathing and diaphragmatic breathing as tools to manage and control feelings of helplessness. He works with patients undergoing rehabilitation for heart disease as well as COPD. Dr. Paluba is the Director of the Stress Management Progam at the Heart Center of St. Francis Hospital in Roslyn, New York and holds clinical and teaching appointments at the Psychoanalytic Center for Communicative Education and the Mt. Sinai School of Medicine, in addition to his private practice.

Editorial

Rivka Arieli, of Vancouver BC, Canada, is a writer of stories whose professional life is focused on writing, editing, and production of technical documentation for major international clients. As editor, she has here melded the work of several individuals while allowing each to speak with his or her unique voice. Rivka has enabled us to speak directly to the reader who has COPD, and transformed the information and emotions into an experience that we hope will give the reader a new lease on life.

Robert Lehr of Lehr Information Services provided editorial production services, informed by professional expertise in physiology.

Jerry Halberstadt was the senior editor.

Design

The page layout and book design is an adaptation of the NTP house style based on advice from David Margolin.

Cover

The cover design is by David Margolin. Special thanks are due to Manuela Paul, an artist and designer who works in Brooklyn and New York City, for her advice and suggestions.

Illustration

The medical illustrations are by Jeanine Theriault. Ms. Theriault is a freelance medical and scientific illustrator. She received her BFA in medical illustration at the Rochester Institute of Technology, and her studios are at Marstons Mills on Cape Cod and Cambridge, Massachusetts. The crucial task of adding labels to illustrations and converting photographs and drawings to electronic form was carried out by Chris Zarza and his staff, including Matt Brown, at Studio Z in Lowell, Massachusetts.

Bulletin board

The HealthyResources bulletin board enabled the authors, editors, and other contributors to collaborate online on the development of this book. Ari Halberstadt created this sophisticated facility, which will be used at <http://www.HealthyResources.com> to enable people with COPD to share information and support. Ari, a skilled nature photographer, also scanned a number of illustrations for this book.

Corporate assistance

Several companies provided information, advice, and the right to use copyrighted material and illustrations. The authors and publisher are grateful for this assistance which was given without conditions affecting editorial content. The inclusion of a product does not represent an endorsement, nor does omission imply any negative evaluation.

Credits for illustrations and source material

The following photographs of Jo-Von Tucker are © 1999 Jerry Halberstadt: *cover*; *Jo-Von Tucker at Clambake Celebrations* on page 17; *Using a metered-dose inhaler* on page 66; *Very small portable container and carrying case* on page 93; *Nasal cannula for delivering oxygen* on page 96; *Pulsed oxygen delivery with nasal cannula* on page 98.

Spirometry testing on page 58; spirometry testing with the QRS SpiroCard PC Card Spirometer, adapted from QRS photo.

Hand-held nebulizer on page 67 shows the Invacare Corporation's Invacare® Passport® Deluxe and Scout® Ultrasonic Nebulizer.

Portable liquid oxygen on page 89; courtesy Mallincrodt—Nellcor Puritan Bennett.

Oxygen concentrator that refills portable cylinders on page 90; Total O2® Delivery System, courtesy CHAD.

Combinations of oxygen systems on page 94; courtesy Mallincrodt—Nellcor Puritan Bennett.

Portable stroller for oxygen on page 93; photo of Jo-Von Tucker © 1998 Frank Bumpus.

Oxygen-conserving nasal cannula on page 98; based on Oxymizer® pendant by CHAD.

Pulsed oxygen delivery with nasal cannula on page 98; Oxylite® system shown courtesy of Cape & Islands Oxygen Supply

Transtracheal oxygen delivery on page 100; SCOOP® transtracheal oxygen, courtesy of Transtracheal Systems.

CPAP and bi-level positive airway pressure devices on page 118; CPAP and bi-level devices and masks courtesy of ResMed, Mallincrodt Nellcor Puritan Bennett, and Sunrise Medical/DeVilbiss.

Cover of the *Brochure* on page 158, courtesy the Cape COPD Support Group.

At a meeting of the Cape Cod COPD Support Group on page 159; Cape COPD Support Group ©1998 Francis Birch.

Before and after lung volume reduction surgery on page 187; Illustrations of lung volume reduction surgery courtesy Julie E. Takasugi, M.D., Department of Radiology, Puget Sound VA Health Care System, 1660 S. Columbian Way, Seattle WA 98108

Respiratory support with a non-invasive ventilator on page 190; Photo showing Respironics BiPAP® device used for respiratory support in hospital, courtesy of Respironics. BiPAP® is a registered mark of Respironics, Inc.

Respirator to provide life support on page 191; Siemens Servo 300A ventilator with AutoMode™ and the Siemens INFINITY™ SC 8000 patient status monitoring system. Illustration courtesy Siemens Medical Systems, Inc., Electromedical Division.

Copyrights and Trademarks

The names of a number of medications, products, and services mentioned in the book may be trademarks, registered marks, or service marks of their respective owners, and they have been so identified at the first use in the book.

The *Nutrition checklist* on page 143 is the "Determine Your Nutrition Health Checklist," of the Nutrition Screening Initiative; and is reprinted with permission by the Nutrition Screening Initiative, a project of the American Academy of Family Physicians, the American Dietetic Association, and the National Council on the Aging, Inc., and funded in part by a grant from Ross Products Division, Abbott Laboratories, Inc.

The motto of the American Lung Association, "If You Can't Breathe, Nothing Else Matters,®" is a registered trademark of the American Lung Association and is used here with permission.

Index

A

abdomen 35
abnormal
    breathing 56
    breathing sounds 56
    large heart 56
absence of alpha-1 antitrypsin 49
acceptance
    stages of 9
action
    of carbon dioxide 37
    of heart 37
    of oxygen 37
active people
    and portable oxygen 92
activities 165
    alternatives 172
    driving 171
    entertaining guests 170
    gardening and yard work 170
    house cleaning 167
    Jo-Von's 172
    less active 165
    meal planning 168
    meal preparation 168
    more active 165
    shopping 167
acupuncture 111
acute respiratory failure 183
addiction
    cigarettes 108
    compulsion and 108
    drug dependence and 108
    World Health Organization
        definition of 108

cigarettes. *See* smoking, stopping
    smoking
adrenaline and isoproterenol 70
advance directives 195, 203
    and state laws 195
    and traveling 196
    storage of 196
advantages
    of conserving devices 99
    of two-function concentrator
        90
aerobic training
    example 134
Aerobid M 72
afford. *See* costs
agreements
    getting a bid 101
    maintenance & alternatives
        101
AIDS 208
air flow difficulty
    COPD 3
air pollution 45, 51
air pressure, sensing changes 97
air travel *See* traveling
air/blood interface 37
airflow, measuring xviii
airway 32
    healthy and diseased 53
airway obstruction
    asthmatic bronchitis 53
    bronchitis 53
    diseases compared 50
    emphysema 53
    overlap of COPD
        components 49
alarms
    and oxygen equipment 89
albuterol 30, 70, 201
alcohol 112
    and mood depression 204
allergic reaction 76
allergy 50
alpha-1 antitrypsin 39
    lack of 49, 53
alpha-1 antitrypsin deficiency
    emphysema 41
    symptoms 50

alternative service agreements
    101
altitude 38
    and extra oxygen 39
aluminum cylinders 91
Alupent 70
alveolar destruction 52
alveolar macrophage 39
alveolar sacs 32
alveoli 32, 34
    damaged 34
    emphysemic 35, 42
    healthy 35, 37, 42
    inflated 34
American Cancer Society 113
American Heart Association 113
American Lung Association 113
    emergency cards 44
    of Hennepin County 171
    of Massachusetts 155
anabolic steroids 71
anesthesia, local
    during tests 60
anger. *See* rage
angina 110
ankle swelling 147
anti-allergy treatment 52
anti-bacterial soap 45
antibiotics 75
    costs 76
    dosages 76
antibodies 39
anti-cholenergic bronchodilators
    70
antifungals 76
antihypertensive medications
    sexual problems and 119
anti-inflammatory
    medications 73
    pills 74
anti-oxidants 206
antivirals 76
anxiety 51, 70, 81
    and breathing 43
    and depression 43
    and fear of death 210
    and feeling helpless 210
    and loss of control 210

and need for oxygen 43
and sense of mortality 210
and thoughts of death 209
as distraction from healing
efforts 209
attack 42
avoiding 42
breathing to control 43
controlling 42
dyspnea as source of 210
feeling helpless 43
from life situation 210
meditation to control 209
overcoming 210
psychological perspective on
210
with Theophylline 75
anxiety attack
and shortness of breath 43
applicators for medications
types of 64
appointments 23
length of 22
arterial blood gases
See oximetry
arterial puncture & pain 60
arteries 36
asbestos 56
asthma 49
airway obstructed 53
symptoms 50
asthmatic bronchitis 41
diagnosis 51
symptoms 50
atmospheric pressure 38
Atrovent 74, 201
Atrovent/atropina 70
attitude 13
availability
of bronchodilators 71
avoidable disease 11
Ayr 156, 203
Azmacort 72

B

back pack 92
back pressure 45
backbone 35
backup
recommendations 91
systems 90
bacteria 39
pneumococcus 77
resistant 76
bad day 59
bad taste 64
balance
of blood gases 36
barometric pressure 38
beclomethasone 72, 74

Beclovent 72
Beconase 74
Beconase AQ 74
behavior modification 110
Beijing Flu 77
benefits
of extra oxygen 85
of stopping smoking 3
beta blockers 55
beta receptor 69
beta-agonist bronchodilators
medium/long acting 70
quick-acting 69
beta-agonists 55
Better Breathers Club 10
bi-level positive airway pressure
as treatment for sleep apnea
117
respiratory support 189
benefits of masks 190
drawbacks of masks 190
BiPAP. *See* bi-level positive
airway pressure
bitolterol 70
bleach solution 68
blocked nasal passages 74
blood
in mucus, urine, bowel
movement 44
vessels 34
blood gas testing 60
reducing pain 60
blood gases
balancing 36
blood pressure
arterioles and 128
circulation and 128
diastolic 60
elevated, and 128
lowering 76
systolic 60
testing 60
up 73
blue fingernails 56
body composition 130
body fat 129
body fat measurement 221
bone loss 71
brain
signals to 38
brain cells
and oxygen deprivation 12
brain damage 13
breastbone 35
breathing 35
abnormal 56
abnormal sounds 56
and anxiety 43
changes in xv, 38
good/bad habits 44
pursed-lip 45

pursed-lip and diaphragmatic
42
rules 45
signals to change 38
tests 57
the system 31
breathing equipment 193
See also oxygen, storage systems,
respiratory support,
obstructive sleep apnea,
CPAP, bi-level positive
airway pressure device
breathless 50
Brethaire 70
bronchi 32
bronchial tubes
bronchitis 32
healthy 32
lining 32
shape of 32
bronchiectasis 49
symptoms 50
bronchioles 32
bronchitis
airway obstructed 53
chronic or asthmatic 41
COPD component 3
symptoms 50
See also chronic bronchitis
bronchodilator 199
bronchodilators 69
anti-cholenergic 70
availability 71
beta-agonist medium/long
acting 70
beta-agonist quick-acting 69
quick acting 30
quick/long acting 42
bronchospasm 55
stopping 73
Bronkometer 70
budesonide 72
bupropion, smoking cessation
and 111
bus exhaust fumes 178

C

cadmium 53
caffeine 112
calorie 144
cancer 105, 208
predictability 4
See also lung cancer 4
canisters. *See* cylinders
cannulas
nasal 96, 97
versus mask 99
capacities
liquid oxygen 88
of composite, steel 92

My Personal Notes and Questions for My Doctor

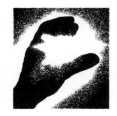

NEW TECHNOLOGY PUBLISHING, INC.

HEALTHY RESOURCES ™

6 West Boulevard, POB 1737, Onset MA 02558 USA
Telephone: 1-888/706-COPD   508/291-1111; 800-672-7632 FAX: 508/291-1704; 800/452-7632
<COPD@newtechpub.com>   <www.HealthyResources.com>   <www.newtechpub.com>

Registration for Healthy Resources

Healthy Resources™ provides access to discussions and support among people with COPD, news and information, and products. <http://www.HealthyResources.com>

This coupon, demonstrating your purchase of *Courage and Information* entitles you to registration and to access the basic individual/family level of services. *Healthy Resources*™ is a service provided by New Technology Publishing, Inc.

Please complete this form and mail to:
New Technology Publishing, Inc., POB 1737 Onset MA 02558 USA
More information: <www.HealthyResources.com>

Name	
Job Title[a]	
Institution/Office	
Address	
Address	
City	
State, Zip	
Office Phone	
Home Phone	
email	
Where did you purchase your copy of *Courage and Information?*	Gift — Online from New Technology — Mail from New Technology — Bookstore — Online Book Store — Health Care Provider — Home Care Provider — Other:_____
Your New Technology Publishing Invoice Number or Sales Receipt Number	

a. Job Title, Institution information only for company orders shipped to your office address, please.

Courage and Information Order Form

To order additional copies of *Courage and Information for Life with Chronic Obstructive Pulmonary Disease* (ISBN 1-882431-07-3, $29.95) direct from the publisher at the special prepaid price (saves $5.00), please complete this form and mail with check or money order to:

New Technology Publishing, Inc., POB 1737 Onset MA 02558 USA

Only on orders shipped to an address in Massachusetts, please add 5% sales tax.

Please write or call 1-888/706-COPD for corporate/institutional orders.

More information: <www.HealthyResources.com>

Online registration: <www.HealthyResources.com/copd/register-book>

Name		List price	$29.95
Job Title[a]		Price with coupon, only	$24.95
Institution/Office		Mass. sales tax	$1.25
Address		Shipping in USA	$5.00
Address		TOTAL	$29.95
City		TOTAL: MA RESIDENTS	$31.20
State, Zip			
Office Phone			
Home Phone			
email			

Ship To Address: Fill out ONLY if different

Name	
Job Title[b]	
Institution/Office	
Address	
Address	
City	
State, Zip	
Office Phone	
Home Phone	
email	

Healthy Resources™ provides access to discussions and support among people with COPD, news and information, and products. <http://www.HealthyResources.com>

Purchase of *Courage and Information* entitles you to registration and to access the basic level of services. *Healthy Resources*™ is a service provided by New Technology Publishing, Inc.

a. Job Title, Institution information only for company orders shipped to office address, please.
b. Job Title, Institution information only for company orders shipped to office address, please.

Family Matters

Collaboration for Health

By Richard Knowles, Ph.D. and Brian L Tiep, M.D.

If a member of your family has COPD, you also have a problem. So, let us address the problem directly. How you and your loved one living with COPD deal with this situation will determine the quality of life for everyone in your family, or if you are living together, in the household. Working together as a family to manage COPD can be an enriching experience. We will try to guide you to a favorable outcome based on our experience in working with many families.

You and your family member with COPD may be fearful of, or already experiencing, a traumatic ordeal. However, no matter how bad the situation may seem to you, the outcome can be much better than you would have imagined.

The person living with COPD is faced with constant breathlessness and a host of physical, financial, and emotional challenges. Panic, anxiety, hopelessness, anger, and depression are only some of the emotions that the person with COPD may experience.

You and other family members are bound to have a wide range of concerns and feelings in response, generated by your love and concern. Thus, you and the other members of the family are also confronted with difficulties. This can lead to an unpleasant emotional roller coaster.

---

1. This Section is addressed to the families of people with COPD; it was first published in the Internet magazine, *COPD TODAY* at www.HealthyResources.com/ Please visit!

There are answers to your questions and concerns. You can learn how the physical and emotional challenges can be met by the person with COPD. You can learn constructive ways for you and other family members to provide help and support to the person with COPD. And your family can work together through the use of clear but sensitive communication.

How your loved one deals with this situation can vary greatly. It is important for you to understand the impact COPD has on your loved one because it impacts your life radically.

It will be up to all parties concerned whether this impact is positive or negative. You might fear that such a set of negative factors would lead to a negative atmosphere within your home. However, by embracing an understanding, creative, and cooperative approach, your family can be enriched by everyone rising to the challenges imposed by COPD.

Frequently Asked Questions:

Here are answers to questions that may provide insight for you as a family:

What is COPD? Can this disease be controlled? What is the outcome?

It means that the person has a Chronic Obstructive Pulmonary (Lung) Disease. The key word are chronic and obstructive. Chronic means that it not curable, but it is certainly manageable. Obstructive means that it is hard to breathe though constricted air passages. This contributes to shortness of breath. COPD is a combination of emphysema, chronic bronchitis and even some asthma. This sounds like we are handing out more disease. In reality, this is a way of understanding and managing a disease with multiple components. It means that there are more opportunities to bring the illness under control.

It is important that the person with COPD have been given a correct diagnosis and has a doctor who fully understands the illness and its total impact upon the family as well as on the person living with COPD. Being short of breath and having the fear of not being able to catch one's breath can raise the tension within the family. There are many ways to relieve shortness of breath and to deal with the emotions surrounding the symptoms of COPD. When the person with COPD is able to understand and to manage the emotional issues as well as the physical symptoms, there will be less stress for the family. Such proven methods of self management can help bring emotional balance back to the family. The person with COPD may ask such questions as: What is self-management? How can this help? What about my doctor? Will he still help me?

How does COPD affect the family of the person living with COPD?

The impact of COPD on the family depends on many factors: the personality of the patient, of family members, and the family structure. COPD can create changes in the family structure, but these changes can be an opportunity for strengthening the family.

Both patient and family may be sharing a ride on an emotional roller coaster. This is a dynamic process that is likely to change over time—without prior notice.

Watch for these emotional pitfalls: anxiety, depression, anger and a cycle of frustration that rapidly spreads across your entire family. How you and your loved one deals with this situation will determine the quality of life for everyone in your house.

Some signs of these pitfalls: sleeping in/ sleeping late; staying up all night; not eating; overeating; lack of communication; too much communication; not dressing, not grooming. Recognize them for what they are—signs of needing help. Don't be judgemental, do be helpful. Be positive and supportive. At some point you may need to get in touch with professional help—start with the doctor caring for the person with COPD; this doctor can best guide you to a referral to a mental health professional. You will want to find a problem-solving professional who will help you sort out these problems and help you find a solution. The ideal professional will know about COPD and chronic illness and have experience in family counselling as well as appropriate professional credentials.

What is the best way to care for a person with COPD?

Both patient and family need an effective approach to managing this disease. We have come up with an acronym for COPD that may help. COPD is: Co-Operation of Patient and Doctor. This implies disease control where the patient's role is to do good daily management; the doctor's role is to direct; and the family's role is to provide support and encouragement. This is a truly co-operative effort! By this method, patients and their families can enjoy a more normal and fulfilling life in spite of this disease.

How does a family member provide support, while encouraging or enabling independence?

Functional and symptom relief come from an understanding of the disease process and the prescribed treatment by the doctor. Emotional relief and support comes from such understanding and empathy. You can learn about COPD and treatments for it, and you can help to educate your loved one who has COPD.

How can I help my loved one who has COPD—didn't they bring this on themselves by years of smoking?

Blame, guilt, anger, and despair may be natural responses when a loved one is sick. We fear losing them and at the same time we may blame them for causing their own disease. These feelings need to be discussed openly and a way found to move past blame and guilt. Some perspective on smoking may help. Smoking is not simply personal choice. It is heavily influenced by tobacco advertising and social pressure and smoking itself is an addiction that is one of the most powerful known to human kind. Smokers are more victims than people making free choices. Not so long ago, more people smoked than not. Those who have quit have overcome major hurdles in detox and habit reshaping. Although most COPD is caused by smoking, it can also be caused by exposure to certain chemicals or be the result of an inherited lack of alpha-one antitrypsin, normally made by the body to help protect the lungs.

Finally, if you grew up in a home with smoking, and/or if you yourself smoked, you can find out if you have any COPD. Your doctor can get you a spirometry test which only requires you to breathe into a test device. The earlier COPD is detected, the sooner you can stop the damage and save your lungs. If you do smoke, you need to think about stopping for your own sake as well as for your family members.

What can be done in the home or automobile to improve COPD?

Maintain a healthy-air household. There should be no smoking, incense, perfumes, or paint fumes. The filters in heating and cooling systems must be changed on a regular basis - often monthly. During times when there is extensive use of heating and air conditioning, the resulting dry air should be humidified.

Don't forget that the car is an enclosed environment that demands an even higher level of care. Avoid being out during high levels of air pollution.

What can we do when everyone is angry, upset, or in a panic?

Perhaps a better way to look at this is to avoid getting into that kind of situation. You should ask, "What can be done to keep the COPD from getting worse?" There should be open and honest discussion of how to deal with the underlying illness as well as the emergencies that are likely to emerge frequently. Set up a partnership and plan with the doctor to help prevent disease progression, avoid emergencies, and effectively avert exacerbations (a worsening of the disease) through early detection and a rapid action plan.

Let's Make the Most of Our Time In an Imperfect World

An Open Letter to Family Members from Your COPD Person—Jo-Von Tucker

Dear Family,

Our lives may never be quite the same, A.D. (after diagnosis). In a perfect world, I wouldn't have COPD. But we can both try to seek more joy, derive more pleasure, from what we are fortunate enough to have... one another. Let's make the most of our time.

In a perfect world, you wouldn't have to wonder how I was feeling, and wonder what you might be able to do to help me. You wouldn't find yourself on the receiving end of my reactions to the episodic depression spells to which I am prone. Nor would you have to puzzle over the fact that I seem to have good days, and then inexplicably, so many bad days.

You must be terribly disturbed by my shortness of breath, and by the fatigue that nibbles at me all day, every day. And I can guess that you are as upset and embarrassed as I am by the fits of coughing that sometimes seize me, especially out in public.

You know that the compromises to my lifestyle that are demanded of me are upsetting. It's hard for me to ask for help, when I find that I can no longer do something on my own. It hurts my pride, and I can see in your eyes that it hurts you, too.

But it isn't a perfect world, is it? I do have this disease, and so far there is no cure for it. I must learn to cope with it. We all must. So, even though the world is less than perfect, particularly so since my diagnosis with chronic lung disease, these issues do exist. I want to find a way to help you as you try to help me.

That's why I'm writing this letter to you now. Sometimes it's just easier to write things down than it is to say them out loud. Especially things that cause this big lump in my throat, even as I write.

You are my loved and cherished family. And it seems to me that the family members are often hit as hard with the realities of COPD as the patient. Maybe even harder. It pains me to see you struggle with solutions for us as we fight the battle of illness together. I know you want to help.

So here is my fantasy of what our nearly perfect world can be, in spite of COPD:

Our lives cannot help but be affected by the fact that I have this disease. But I have learned that COPD is not a death sentence... nor does it have to be the end of our quality of life. The better I become at managing my own illness, the more effective and happier our time together will be. Maybe if we establish some suggested ground rules to get us through the rough patches, we'll adapt more easily and with less stress on us all. Here's my list of seven suggestions:

Suggestion #1: It is important for me to remain as independent as possible to preserve my self-esteem. Try not to rush to help me before you know whether or not I can accomplish a task on my own. I really want to try; not only to spare you, but also to help me with my independence and self esteem, both of which will erode significantly with every thing that I learn I can't do.

There is a fine line that you, my dear ones, must walk in balancing between coming to my aid, or just taking over for me, (which can be interpreted as enabling me to become a cripple). This is important for so many reasons, like the need to keep my body and muscles as conditioned and toned as is humanly possible under these circumstances. Like the need that I have to feel useful, again—to help guard against a loss of self esteem.

Suggestion #2: Try to not judge me if I'm having a bad day. It is possible that a lung infection could be brewing in my body, and you may be aware of it sooner than I can be myself. You know the signs... increased shortness of breath and coughing up discolored sputum. Perhaps fever, but maybe not. Less energy to expend on the simple chores of daily living.

Some of the folks in my lung support group have expressed their frustration when their family leaps to the conclusion that we are hypochondriacs who complain a lot about feeling bad. I think that this just isn't so; we aren't constant complainers. The COPDers I've come to know are a pretty brave lot, all in all. Most of us who have some form of COPD do not want our loved ones to see us as "sickly" or making excuses. As a result, however, many of us hedge about the problems we are having.

Suggestion #3: Please help me by overseeing that I am complying with my doctor's prescribed treatment plan. I don't expect you to be a nurse, but I will appreciate it if you gently remind me to take my afternoon puffs on my inhalers, or to check to see if I remembered to take my evening pills.

Help me to be a compliant patient by helping with my oxygen equipment when we go out. It's good to know that I have a portable filled with enough supplemental oxygen to get me comfortably through our schedule. It's also good to have help getting in and out of the car. And especially helpful to have an arm to lean on going up stairs, if I need it. The more comfortable we both are with the oxygen and equipment that I need, the sooner it will be accepted and not questioned by the general public.

Suggestion #4: Help me to stay socialized. Do not let me become isolated from friends and other family members. We COPD folks do have a tendency to stay at home, rather than digging down deep for the energy to get up and out! You can encourage me to accompany you to lunch, or even to the market. You can inspire me to go to a movie, or to have guests in for bridge, scrabble or cribbage. Your encouragement can make the difference for me---desiring to see people, and for people to see me!

Suggestion #5: In this nearly perfect world, we need to have and show respect for one another. I promise that I won't talk about you as if you aren't in the room, if you'll do the same for me. My feelings are currently worn very close to the surface; I can hear perfectly well what you've said to someone about how fast the disease is progressing, or about how futile our efforts to fight it may seem. You and I can certainly discuss these issues between ourselves, and keep them within the family circle.

Suggestion #6: Encourage me (but please don't nag me) about getting my exercises in each day. Some days it is just so hard to commit to even 10 minutes of active exercises. If I'm too sick to do them myself, try to help me with just some stretching exercises like yoga or T'ai Chi. These gentle movements can help to keep my body conditioned, even when I'm suffering from an exacerbation. And they aren't that taxing of my strength or energy. You, of course, no matter how hard you try, can not fully understand how I am feeling because you don't have my lung disease. But your encouragement brings me added strength; your emotional support brings me peace from the trauma of being sick.

Suggestion #7 Nutrition is an important part of helping my body with its special needs. You can help by making sure that I'm eating right. A diet high in protein will help build up my immune system and body strength. We can plan the week's menus together. I pledge to try and tell you what items seem to taste best to me.

That's it... I'll stop with Lucky #7. I don't wish to make our lives more difficult with suggestions and rules. I simply want to express myself on the subject of how you can help me. I don't want to sound as though I am whining or complaining. I am reaching out with all the love that is in my heart for the help that I know you want to provide. And if you have your own list of suggestions, please share them with me.

It is true that our lives may never be quite the same. But we can work together to preserve and enhance what we are fortunate enough to have... one another. Help me to continue to fight on, to become stable, to endure what I will not let bring me down. Let's make the most of our time.

From my heart to yours,

Your Person with COPD, Jo-Von Tucker